# Life Without Arthritis

*The Maori Way*

## A REMARKABLE DISCOVERY FOR ARTHRITIS AND RHEUMATISM SUFFERERS

# Jan de Vries

MAINSTREAM
PUBLISHING

EDINBURGH AND LONDON

First published in 1991 by
MAINSTREAM PUBLISHING COMPANY (EDINBURGH) LTD
7 Albany Street
Edinburgh EH1 3UG

Reprinted 1995, 1999

A catalogue record for this book is available from the British Library

ISBN 1 85158 471 4 (cased)
1 85158 466 8 (paperback)

Typeset in 11/12 Palatino
Reproduced from disc by Polyprint, 48 Pleasance, Edinburgh, EH8 9TJ
Printed and bound in Finland by WSOY

# LIFE WITHOUT ARTHRITIS THE MAORI WAY

To people in the West the name 'Maori' conjures up images of a tribal society. Not quite so widely known, however, is the fact that this race tends to live to a great age — by and large unhampered by ill-health or the traditional diseases now accepted by us as being an unavoidable consequence of growing old. For even among the Maori elders there is usually no sign of rheumatism or arthritis. Indeed, there is little evidence to suggest that these conditions have ever existed in their culture.

In *Life Without Arthritis* Jan de Vries shows how the dietary management of the Maori people is the major source of continued good health — and that it is a diet now widely available in Western society. He shares the treasures of the Maoris and explains how, by following their example, there *can* be life without arthritis or rheumatism.

Books available from the same author in the
By Appointment Only series:

*Stress and Nervous Disorders* (sixth edition)

*Multiple Sclerosis* (third edition)

*Traditional Home and Herbal Remedies* (fourth edition)

*Arthritis, Rheumatism and Psoriasis* (fifth edition)

*Do Miracles Exist?*

*Neck and Back Problems* (fifth edition)

*Migraine and Epilepsy* (fourth edition)

*Cancer and Leukaemia* (second edition)

*Viruses, Allergies and the Immune System* (fourth edition)

*Realistic Weight Control*

*Heart and Blood Circulatory Problems*

*Asthma and Bronchitis*


Books available from the same author in the
Nature's Gift series:

*Body Energy*

*Water — Healer or Poison?*


Also available from the same author:

*Who's Next?*

# Contents

*Honoe te pito ora ki te pito pate.*

*(Let the strong end be joined to the weak end —* Maori proverb)

# 1

## The Maoris

ON 1 APRIL 1970 we opened our residential clinic on the west coast of Scotland, called Mokoia. It was housed in a beautiful mansion overlooking the Clyde and the Isle of Arran, beyond which the Irish Sea could be seen. I doubt if anybody could express in words the beauty and full glory of a sunset viewed from Mokoia and do it justice.

When I opened the clinic in Scotland, I was ignorant of the meaning of the name. I asked around and checked with libraries, but I didn't really know where to start. What did the name "Mokoia" mean? From various sources I was given different interpretations. The explanation I liked the best originated in New Zealand and related to an island in the New Zealand lake district which, according to Maori legend, was often referred to as "the Island of Love".

This legend comes to us from the unwritten records of a highly cultured people. The island of Mokoia is surrounded by a lake in Rotorua, an area that is famous for its thermal lakes and is steeped in legend, history and culture. Rotorua is a land of romance. Every hill and valley, every geyser and boiling mud pool, every lake and island and indentation of the shore was known by name and loved by the Maori people. Many of these places were immortalised in fable and story, and this is not surprising. A region of violent thermal activity is an obvious setting for tales of mystery and magic, many of which have been handed down from the distant past.

"*I kapi i be cangata*", the Maoris used to say of the island of Mokoia, which means "covered with men". It is only a small island, about one mile square, rising in proud isolation 500 feet above the level of the lake and protected by its waters. It has a history that can be traced back more than a thousand years. The island of Mokoia was originally inhabited by an indigenous tribe who were conquered by the Arawa people. *Te arawa* means "the canoe". About six centuries ago some of the more adventurous people from Tahiti set out on exploratory journeys: in a fleet of canoes they sailed southwards, where they eventually settled at Maketu in the Bay of Plenty. From there the Arawa people spread inland and eventually conquered the indigenous tribes of the Hot Lakes district — the guardians of the fascinating thermal region of New Zealand. It is in this area that the island of Mokoia is to be found.

In their legends we read about Ngatoro — "the fire-bringer". It is claimed that upon finding dry valleys he stamped his foot so hard that springs of water gushed forth. It was Ngatoro who first visited the mountains and placed on them the mysterious white-skinned fairy people; legend also had it that it was Ngatoro who was the cause of volcanic fire, spouting geysers and boiling mud pools.

The early name of Mokoia was *Te Mokotapu-a-Tinirau*, meaning "the Sacred Isle of Tiniran". Its later name, Mokoia, is a curious example of a native pun. Many years went by before the original inhabitants were finally exterminated or absorbed by the Arawa tribe. One of these aboriginals was Arorangi, a tribal chief, who had killed and eaten a dog belonging to an Arawa chief. As a result, a battle was fought and Arorangi was killed by the Arawa chief. He was struck over the eye with the sharp point of a *ko*, which is a digging implement. The wound was made where his face was closely tattooed. When news of this spread, it was referred to as the battle of Mokoia, which means tattooed, and is also a play on the words *moko* (tattooed) and *ko* (digging implement). The name of the battle was afterwards transferred to the island.

One of the many things for which the island was noted was the kumara god to be found there. The *kumara* is a type of sweet potato which formed part of the Maoris' staple diet. The kumara god was portrayed on a stone emblem and venerated as the god of fertility. It stood about four feet high and was brought over to Mokoia by an Arawa canoe. For many years the stone emblem was kept in a tiny wooden building, which could almost be described as a miniature temple. In the planting season the tribes of the district would make a pilgrimage to Mokoia, carrying seed-kumara. They would touch the sacred effigy with the seed to ensure the fertility of their crop. In the warm, volcanic soil the god protected the plantations against blight and frost. *"Kia tu tangatanga te aro ki Mokoia"* ("Let the way be open to Mokoia") was a local saying which recognised the power of the kumara god.

In the year 1823 the islanders suffered severe losses against a northern tribe led by the redoubtable chief

9

Hongi Hika. At this time Hongi was the most feared man in New Zealand. Three years earlier he had set sail for Britain, where King George IV granted him an audience and presented him with a suit of armour, among other gifts. At Sydney, on his way back to New Zealand, he exchanged many of these presents for muskets and ammunition, and on his arrival at the Bay of Islands he lost no time in achieving his ambition — becoming overlord of all the tribes. The local tribes were helpless against warriors who were armed with the weapons of the white man, and Hongi's raids became a bloody procession of victories. It was in the early part of 1823 that Hongi set out with a flotilla of canoes and an army of bloodthirsty fighting men to subdue the Arawa.

The people of Rotorua, aware that Hongi would have to march overland to reach their settlement, considered themselves impregnable in the fortress of Mokoia, with the vast moat of the lake as their protection. But Hongi was better armed and more cunning than his opponents. His canoes were paddled up the river and then hauled overland, from where he reached the lake. Early one morning, while the mists still lay heavy on the lake, the Arawa tribe slept peacefully. The sentries were on watch, but could see nothing through the mist. Suddenly, the Arawa people were alerted as the gulls screamed overhead and they rushed to defend the beaches. Ever since that ill-fated morning, the watchful gulls of Mokoia have been held in reverence by the Arawa tribe, who will allow no one, Maori or white man, to molest the sacred birds, in whose bodies, they say, still live the spirits of warriors who died in battle.

Hongi was cunning and for three days his canoes encircled the island. A few of the Arawa people managed to escape by swimming to the mainland by night. Then came the time that Hongi's men opened fire and made their bridgehead on the northern shore, from where their guns were used to mow down the opposition. From that point they soon gained possession of the whole island, although many lives were lost on both sides. Eventually, a truce was negotiated between Hongi and the Arawa chief and Hongi returned home, taking many prisoners with him.

With some knowledge of the history of the island of Mokoia you may be able to appreciate the fantastic legends of its people so much better. One of their best-known and best-loved legends is the love story of Hinemoa.

The young chief Tutanekai lived with his parents on the island. On a tribal visit to the lakeside village of Owhata, Tutanekai saw and promptly fell in love with the beautiful young chieftainess of Owhata. Young women of Hinemoa's status were closely guarded and Tutanekai had no opportunity of telling her of his love when it was time for him to return to the island of Mokoia.

Hinemoa had seen the way that this young man had looked at her and, although he had not been able to express his intentions, she had understood. Each night, as the story tells us, Tutanekai stood on the verandah, thinking of Hinemoa. He would play his nose-flute, hoping that his message would find its way to Hinemoa's heart. The days and nights dragged slowly, until at last another visit was made to Owhata by the tribe of Mokoia.

While the dancers of Owhata entertained their guests, the lovers stood outside in the shadows. Hinemoa promised her suitor that she would come to him, but warned him that she had to come alone, without telling anyone. Then she asked, "How shall I know when you will be ready?"

Tutanekai promised that the next evening he would again play the flute and when she heard the music she was to come quietly down to the beach, take a small canoe and paddle across the lake, where he would be waiting for her.

The next evening, when Hinemoa heard the music, she crept down to the beach, only to find that all the canoes had been pulled well up the beach, behind protective boulders and into the bush. She did not have sufficient strength to drag even the smallest canoe across the boulders. Sadly, she returned to her sleeping house. The next night she hurried down in the darkness once again, but the canoes were still out of reach. She then knew that her plans had been suspected, for some of the canoes had been used during the day and they would not normally have been pulled up into the bush.

Night after night went by and her heart seemed to call out in desperation as she heard the flute's song but could not leave the island. Eventually, she decided to swim to her lover. Secretly, she prepared six empty gourds, tying them together with flax. On the first moonlit night she went down to the beach and tied the gourds firmly round her body. She swam with all the strength and courage she had, listening to the music for her directions, until eventually her knee struck sand. Overcome with relief, she staggered up the beach, half dead with cold. When next she listened, the music had gone, for it was late and Tutanekai had given up hope.

In the dark Hinemoa felt her way carefully until she touched some rocks which felt strangely warm. There was a smell of sulphur-laden steam and a few moments later she lowered her body cautiously into the luxurious warmth of a hot pool. She knew then where she was, for this was the pool known as Wai-kimihia, which lay directly beneath Tutanekai's hut. As her body gratefully

absorbed the warmth, she became aware of her naked-
ness and felt ashamed. It was then that she heard foot-
steps on the path leading down from her lover's hut
and she hid behind the boulders. Disguising her voice
to sound like a man she asked: "Who are you?"

"I am filling a calabash for my master, Tutanekai,"
came the reply. When she heard this she asked for
the calabash and when the slave passed it to her she
hurled it against the rocks, where it smashed into a
dozen pieces. She then sunk out of sight behind the
rocks. When the slave asked her why she had done
that, he received no answer. He returned to Tutanekai's
hut and confessed to his master what had happened.
Tutanekai had been tossing restlessly on his sleeping mat,
wondering whether Hinemoa had changed her mind.
He instructed the slave to go back and not to drop
the calabash again. At the pool the story repeated itself
and again the slave returned without water to Tutanekai.
Tutanekai sent his slave to the pool a third time, with the
warning that he would regret it if he returned without
water. Meanwhile, dawn was about to break and at the
first sound of the deep, male voice the slave fled back
to his master's hut and told Tutanekai that he was not to
blame.

Tutanekai decided to go and look for himself. "Where
are you, breaker of pots?" he demanded quietly. "Come
out like a man!"

There was no reply, for Hinemoa had sunk down
so deep that her hair floated like seaweed on the still
water. Tutanekai circled the pool until his eyes became
accustomed to the subdued light and then he put down
his hand and grasped her hair. Slowly, Hinemoa stood
upright in the light of early morning, facing her lover
with an uncertain smile. As they embraced, Tutanekai
understood that Hinemoa's love for him was greater than

many waters and that nothing had been able to stop her coming to him.

This lovely old story is still kept very much alive in Maori culture.

I feel a great affinity with the Maori people, particularly because I have been able to give my patients at Mokoia clinic in Scotland some of that health and happiness with which the Maoris were blessed. It was at that same clinic that, one morning, a lady from a neighbouring town came to see me, having recently returned from New Zealand. I had been treating her for many months for rheumatoid arthritis and she had followed my instructions to the letter. She had indeed made some progress, but nowhere near sufficient to even hint at a cure. On this visit, soon after her return from New Zealand, she informed me that she had made the most fantastic recovery while she had been away, and all because she had been introduced to the green-lipped mussel extract. She claimed that this had changed her life and described how this extract, which is obtained from the gonads, or sex glands, of the green-lipped mussel (*Perna canaliculus*) had provided astonishing relief from her pain.

I remembered how gnarled this lady's fingers had been and was amazed to see how they had straightened out. Of course, I was fascinated by her story. I decided to make every effort to find out what was so special about this remedy which, she told me, was gaining great popularity in New Zealand.

All this took place quite a few years ago and since that time I have prescribed the green-lipped mussel extract to many of my patients. Nowadays I regularly prescribe other products in combination with it — always to the benefit of my patients.

We can thank the Maoris for quite a few things and, although their diet is not one of the healthiest, whether or not a diet is balanced is the crucial factor and this could well give us a clue as to why rheumatism was unknown among the Maoris. Could we perhaps learn a lesson from them? I certainly believe so!

Over hundreds of years, before the arrival of white settlers in the nineteenth century, the Maoris created a complex and sophisticated society with a flourishing artistic tradition. However, with the introduction of European diseases, weapons and values, many aspects of Maori traditional culture were degraded.

Nowadays, after more than a century of colonisation, intermarriage, etc., there are still over 300,000 Maoris in New Zealand, accounting for approximately ten per cent of the total population. Given their rich history it is not surprising that the Maoris are eager to reclaim their land, their heritage and their culture. Many of them are involved in a reassessment of their society and they are striving for an opportunity to return to the harmonious, loving way of life they once enjoyed.

The Maoris, who have been strongly influenced by the Polynesian peoples of the Pacific through colonisation and intermarriage, traditionally followed a rural lifestyle. The rapid growth of the population in recent times has created a young society and one that is continuing to grow faster than might have been expected. It is encouraging to see that Maori communities are determined to hold on to their social customs. They have revived communal gatherings for tribal discussion and many old ceremonies and traditions are still maintained. I have great admiration for their efforts to hold on to some of their traditional values, customs and rituals so as to ensure that their heritage will not be lost.

It is also interesting that, traditionally, the Maoris were experts at raising plants like the kumara, or sweet potato; they had a sound understanding of soil conditions and cultivation techniques. Captain Cook was impressed with their fighting abilities, the culture of their tribal civilisation, their self-sufficiency and knowledge of crop cultivation, bird-snaring and fishing. Their diet was heavily reliant on the availability of seafood and this is a recurring theme in their legendary tales and traditions.

Sir George Grey, who was Her Majesty's Governor of New Zealand for two periods during the latter half of the nineteenth century, was awed by the Maoris' sophistication and even considered the Maori chiefs to be a superior race of men. However, as a result of colonisation and its side-effects, Maori society became degraded, demoralised and depressed, while the people's health suffered due to foods introduced by the westerners. Then two young men stepped in, Maui Pomari and Peter Black, who were medical officers and two truly brilliant figures. They were determined to help the Maori people to return to a more natural lifestyle and so regain their health. I am delighted to learn that, according to reports from the New Zealand Department of Health, it is their aim to support the Maori people in their efforts to achieve the highest possible level of well-being. Moreover, the programme that has been drawn up recognises emphatically the holistic philosophy of health traditionally embraced by the Maoris and many other people in the Rotorua area.

The new government-backed health schemes aim to re-establish and strengthen the Maoris' cultural and tribal traditions, and so promote a positive outlook among the younger generation. The Department of Health has made a major step in the right direction by recognising the importance of the *Te Taha Weerua* — spiritual well-being — in its programme and they are also encouraging the Maori people to implement their own health projects.

Originally, the Maoris tended to grill most of their foods and use gourds for preservation. Coastal dwellers were familiar with many kinds of shellfish and would generally eat these raw. The many wild plants provided them with an ample supply of edible fruits, pith, shoots, leaves, fruits, flowers or pollen, and the most important of these was fern root — *aruhe* — which served as the staple food for most Maoris. Aruhe is grown in most areas and can be dug up at any time of the year. The Maoris regarded this root as their most reliable food source, as is clear from one of their proverbs:

"He who digs fern root lives,
While he who sneers, dies. . . ."

Sweet potatoes, taro and yams were cultivated for domestic use, while gourds were also used to provide calabashes, or containers, to hold water. The sweet potato — kumara — grew prolifically in the wild and was also cultivated, and this too was a favourite and important source of food, and one which certainly provided the Maoris with a good intake of minerals and trace elements.

Maori culture has been described as having a complementary or holistic pattern. When we compare the complementary nature of their relationships and methods with those of our own society — with technology constantly reaching new heights of sophistication — we too would be wise to return to nature and learn a lesson from the Maoris. Let us consider how they regained their health and happiness when once it seemed that it was all but lost.

The kumara, or sweet potato, supplied the Maoris with their energy requirements and, together with large quantities of fish, provided them with the strength they needed for the many battles they fought.

17

Another factor is the determination and patience they have displayed in tackling certain problems. Certainly, these have proved formidable characteristics of the Maori people.

By now, you will no doubt be wondering what all this has to do with arthritis. To my mind, what we have learned about the Maori way of life could well provide us with the answer to the question of why the Maoris were unfamiliar with any arthritic or rheumatic conditions. This fact first gave me the impetus to study the Maori lifestyle, the food they ate, the way they prepared their food, the herbs they used and, especially, the significance of their use of mussels. Their appreciation of food does not stem from recent times; from their traditional stories we learn that they were often involved in quarrels over the ownership of food sources, and especially the common mussel, *Perna canaliculus*, which was eaten almost daily.

It was the extract of this same mussel that was brought by my patient to our clinic, Mokoia, in Scotland. And here the coincidence of the similar names seems prophetic, because this mussel extract has brought health and happiness back into the lives of many sufferers of rheumatism and arthritis. Not only can New Zealand claim to be a beautiful and fascinating country with its lakes and geysers, but it can also claim a wealth of historical tradition, and a rich Maori culture. This ancient culture can now be credited with the supply of a food supplement that is beneficial in the treatment of a degenerative disease from which millions of people suffer all over the world. The sheer coincidence of the name Mokoia would at any time be a reason for my close affinity with the Maori people, but the many patients whom I have treated in that clinic with the green-lipped mussel have their own constant reminders of the benefits of this surprising New Zealand remedy.

# 2

## *The Green-lipped Mussel*

THERE ARE MANY different schools of thought and different methods available for the treatment of rheumatism and arthritis. At one time it was thought that acupuncture was the only method one could rely on for help; shortly afterwards it was fashionable to think that osteopathy was the sure way for pain relief. Then we were told that diet was all-important, and then again wearing a copper bracelet was said to be the answer. All these different ideas prove that there is no foolproof way to combat degenerative diseases such as arthritis or rheumatism. Indeed, the treatment will vary according to the patient's individual circumstances.

Researchers state that in Great Britain alone osteoarthritis affects five million men, women and children. Rheumatoid arthritis is estimated to affect one to two million people, and then there are the countless sufferers of psoriatic arthritis. Considering these statistics makes it blatantly obvious that positive action is required to fight these crippling diseases. In each individual case some form of treatment can be found that will prove effective, but different categories of patients will benefit from different forms of treatment. We should realise, however, that with such serious degenerative diseases there is rarely a quick response to effective treatment, which means that patience is necessary.

Every now and then we learn about new discoveries from newspaper articles, or radio or television programmes. The latest, which I heard about while preparing this book, is a report from a group of doctors based at a well-known British hospital, who have been monitoring the conditions of pregnant rheumatoid arthritis patients. The report claims that during pregnancy many women with rheumatism or arthritis experience a remission and that many of the symptoms of the disease disappear altogether. It goes so far as to state that 75 per cent of pregnant women are completely symptom-free.

The improvement appears to be caused by a protein which they have called PAG — Pregnancy Associated Glycoprotein. The report says that PAG "is present in pregnant women in large quantities but it is almost undetectable in non-pregnant women".

The importance of the role played by PAG in pregnant women with rheumatoid arthritis is shown by the fact that the symptoms of the disease usually return almost as soon as the baby is born — usually within six weeks. Research is continuing to see if PAG could prove to be the substance capable of stopping arthritis.

I suspect that since the Maoris lived so much closer to nature, they instinctively knew what was good for them. The green-lipped mussel was considered almost divine and during their tribal festivities it was held in great esteem. The mussel was part of their staple diet,

20

but the green-lipped mussel was considered to be something quite special. How right they were, because it is now widely acknowledged that the green-lipped mussel has anti-inflammatory properties that provide great relief to arthritic patients and those who suffer from related degenerative diseases.

The beneficial remedy obtained from the green-lipped mussel is extracted from the gonads, i.e. the reproductive glands. If we relate this to the hormonal imbalance that can be observed in people suffering from arthritic conditions, it points us to the activity of a tiny gland at the base of the brain, called the pituitary gland. At any sign of stress this gland releases a hormone which sounds the alarm. The hormone travels in the blood until it reaches the adrenals. These are two small glands that sit in our kidneys in the middle of the back. When the adrenals receive this hormone they too release different hormones. The chief of these is called cortisol (we know it as cortisone). Messages also come from the nervous system, resulting in the release of the hormone adrenalin. The presence of these adrenal hormones in the blood tells the whole body that it is under threat.

The body's reaction is dramatic. Sugar reserves pour into the blood for immediate fuel, followed by proteins and fats which in turn are broken down into sugars to provide yet more energy. Calcium is taken from our bones to be used by the nerves and muscles. Pain, stiffness and inflammation miraculously disappear. The blood pressure rises to allow oxygen, sugar and calcium to travel more quickly to the tissues.

This stress reaction is highly protective. Normally, when the threat passes, the above reactions are reversed; proteins are built up again and the cells are repaired, and calcium is drawn back into the bones. The blood pressure drops to its normal level, and all our familiar aches and pains reappear. However, the body's reserves will have been depleted and more will be needed for repairs. More vitamins, minerals, protein, fats and carbohydrates will be needed than usual. At this point, when our nutrition is inadequate, or when the stress situation is prolonged, the body will come under further threat. By robbing Peter to pay Paul, it will naturally do the best it can, for as long as possible. Nevertheless, sooner or later we will find we have no more reserves, we cannot make any more adrenal hormones, and we have no further resistance. Disease is the result.

The removal of calcium from bones under stress is clearly one feature of the arthritic process. Normally, calcium moves continuously between blood and bone to maintain a healthy balance. A hormone from the parathyroid glands in the neck takes calcium from the bones when the blood level drops. Calcitonin, a hormone from the thyroid gland, encourages calcium back to the bones. Vitamins are needed for us to absorb calcium from our food and also to help bones to mineralise.

The balance of calcium is very delicate. If the blood calcium levels drop, our muscles may go into spasm and eventually convulsions may result. If our bones are continuously leached of calcium, they may become fragile and will fracture easily. If the level of blood calcium stays high when the body is under stress, then calcium may be deposited in the arteries, tissues, muscles and joints. This tendency to calcification appears to be an error, resulting from either prolonged stress without adequate nutrition, a parathyroid imbalance or vitamin deficiency.

The adrenals produce cortisol from the hormone deoxy-cortisol (known as DOC for short). This hormone has a remarkable action. It helps the body to fight infection and damage by setting up an inflammation around bacteria or toxins and sealing them off, as in the case of a boil for example. Swelling, pain and fever may result but the body is protected. Normally, sufficient DOC will be converted to cortisol to remove the pain and swelling once the intruder has been dealt with.

When the diet does not supply the vitamins needed by the enzymes that make and balance these hormones, DOC may fail to be converted and the areas of pain and swelling may become permanent and collect calcium. It is important to realise that treatment with cortisone is not the easy solution to this problem. This is because our own DOC production is inhibiting lower resistance, thus the bones will be further demineralised, other mineral reactions will cause water retention (moon face), and the constant robbing of proteins may eat away our stomach cells and cause ulcers.

There are seven endocrine glands in the human body and I have occasionally likened the endocrine system to a musical octave. Although there are eight notes to a musical octave, there are really only seven basic notes. The seven endocrine glands may appear small and insignificant, but it is only when one of them is not functioning correctly that we realise the importance of these small glands. There are also seven colours in the solar spectrum, and the number seven has a further significance as the retina of the eye contains seven layers of light receptors. If the number seven were to be considered as the number of perfection, I would have to point out that with arthritic conditions one should look at the perfection of nature, which often gives a clear indication of what should be done.

The Maoris seemed to have recognised intuitively the beneficial properties of the green-lipped mussel. The reproductive glands are a very important part of the endocrine system, yet it is unlikely that the Maoris knew that the gonads produce prostaglandin in the body. According to the newspaper article that I mentioned at the beginning of this chapter, the glyco-protein is the major factor that holds the answer for many arthritic sufferers.

Clinical trials in New Zealand, as well as double-blind trials in Paris, Glasgow, Toronto, and other parts of the world, have proved that the green-lipped mussel extract encapsulated has highly beneficial properties, especially for arthritic and rheumatic conditions.

It is true that scientists are unsure about *why* the extract should be so effective, but the decrease of the characteristic swellings and nodules, and the straightening of fingers I have observed in patients, cannot be denied. These phenomena have often made me wonder if this remarkable product would also be able to influence the hormonal balance.

One cannot argue with visible results, and the improvement I have seen in patients is sufficient testimony in itself as far as I am concerned. Yet I am pleased that so much clinical research has taken place. There is some evidence that osteoarthritis runs in families and so could be hereditary. Rheumatoid arthritis, on the other hand, could be caused by a virus or an infection. The difference between the two is that osteoarthritis affects the cartilage covering the ends of bones and not the lining of the joints, while rheumatoid arthritis is an inflammation affecting the joints and other body tissues. Whatever the cause or the name of the disease, these painful afflictions merit the full attention of the medical establishment.

It appears that it was only by chance that American researchers discovered that the green-lipped mussel possesses anti-inflammatory properties. This large type of mussel, with a distinctive green shell, is found only off the coast of New Zealand. After its therapeutic properties had been discovered, a New Zealand company realised the potential for using the mussel to treat rheumatic diseases and began to produce the extract in capsule form.

The first evaluation of the extract took place at Otago Medical School in New Zealand in 1974. The capsules were tested in a double-blind cross-over trial on six patients over a period of twelve weeks. No positive effects were noted, but to be statistically valid, the test sample should have been larger. The test period was also too brief, as individual case studies have subsequently shown the need for prolonged treatment of up to six months.

In 1976 a preliminary clinical trial commenced at the Glasgow Homoeopathic Hospital in Scotland. Over a period ranging from three months to three years, forty-six patients suffering from chronic cases of rheumatoid arthritis and ten from osteoarthritis took part. The patients were assessed at regular intervals, using the assessment parameters normally associated with trials involving arthritic patients. The results indicated that 60 per cent of the rheumatoid and 30 per cent of the osteo patients benefited from the mussel extract treatment.

The preliminary study led to a six-month double-blind trial at the Victoria Infirmary and Homoeopathic Hospital in Glasgow in 1980. The trial group this time consisted of twenty-eight patients with clinical rheumatoid arthritis and thirty-eight with clinical and radiological evidence of osteoarthritis. Over a six-month period the patients added either the mussel extract or the placebo capsules to their regular treatment. The published results were similar to those of the longer-term preliminary study: 68 per cent of the rheumatoid and 40 per cent of the osteo patients benefited from the mussel extract treatment.

From 1979 to 1982 a number of universities and hospitals in New Zealand and Australia conducted trials to evaluate the anti-inflammatory properties of the mussel extract. The trials, using animal models, confirmed that the mussel extract possessed a specific anti-inflammatory property, and had a gastro-protective effect. The same researchers repeated the trials with extracts from other shellfish, but found that none shared the properties of the green-lipped mussel.

In 1981, a long-term toxicological study indicated that even at high doses the product had no toxic effects. Separate investigations at the Royal Melbourne Institute of Technology involving biochemical and pharmacological studies concluded that the mussel extract possessed significant anti-inflammatory activity, which appeared to be associated with the non-lipid fractions of the extract.

Clinical trials continued at St Bartholomew's Hospital in London in 1981. Thirty patients with rheumatoid arthritis took part in an eight-week cross-over trial. No specific effects were demonstrated by treatment with the extract, but the results were considered inconclusive. The trial group and period was small and involved a cross-over from mussel extract to placebo after only four weeks.

Subsequent studies were undertaken at Auckland Hospital and the Glasgow Centre for Rheumatic Diseases in 1983, and research also commenced at the University of Shizuoka in Japan. The Japanese study investigated the anti-arthritic activity of the mussel extract by attempting to isolate the active principle, and obtained positive results.

The latest trials commenced in France in 1985, involving over two hundred patients in three separate, double-blind, placebo-controlled trials. The results of the first study on arthritis of the knee have recently been published and they convincingly demonstrate the efficacy of the mussel extract. Reports of the other trials, on osteoarthritis and on patients undergoing radiation therapy, are due to be published at a later date.

Thus, we have ample evidence to conclude that scientific and clinical trials have clearly demonstrated that the green-lipped mussel extract has a therapeutic effect on both rheumatoid and osteo arthritis. The active principle may yet have to be identified, but there is no doubt about its anti-inflammatory properties.

Nowadays, green-lipped mussels are not so readily found on the shores of New Zealand, although they can be purchased from seafood shops having been obtained from marine farms. This appears to be one of the reasons that the contemporary diet of the Maori population no longer regularly includes this nutritional food. Yet another reason is the fact that many Maoris have moved away from their rural and coastal homes to live in the larger cities, where they can find employment more easily. Yet, when obtainable, the mussel still constitutes a popular part of their diet.

The age and size of the green-lipped mussel has now become a matter of availability. The Maoris traditionally prefer large mussels, but these are now very scarce from natural sources and are totally unavailable from farmed stocks. However, farmed stock yields very succulent and tender young mussels and these are becoming increasingly popular.

The Maoris prefer to eat the mussel raw without any preparation at all. However, they also enjoy barbecued mussels where the live shellfish is placed on a hot-plate over a fire and left to cook briefly in its own juices. In earlier times some 80 per cent of the Maori diet used to be seafood, mainly shellfish. The use of mussels other than the green-lipped variety is now virtually unknown. Blue mussels do grow naturally in certain areas of New Zealand, but these are regarded as a nuisance by mussel farmers and they are not marketed domestically.

There is little statistical evidence of an increase in arthritic disorders among Maoris, but the tribal chiefs are convinced that the incidence of arthritis has increased significantly in recent years. Some of the blame may be apportioned to the fact that many Maoris have become city dwellers and will now shop at supermarkets along with everyone else and eat processed and convenience foods. Apart from the really traditional Maori, they eat the same foods as everyone else in New Zealand, including a relatively high proportion of so-called "junk food".

It is claimed that the green-lipped mussel was not knowingly used in native medicine for its therapeutic properties, as the Maoris were unaware of its benefits, but they now readily accept its beneficial actions as they believe in natural medicines provided by nature. The modern-day Maori is not really concerned with the mode of action as this is in the pharmacological field, but they instinctively believe in giving the body the things that will encourage it to help itself.

Other foods eaten by the Maori people were not specifically health-enhancing from a medical point of view. Obviously, their diet — high in seafoods, with plenty of vegetables and only a minimum of red meat — was a healthy one, but was not consciously eaten for prophylactic or remedial purposes. However, the Maoris did make extensive use of certain plants for medicinal purposes.

According to a publication from the *New Zealand Medical Journal* of 10 September 1980:

During the past years there has been an increasing amount of interest in the use of a preparation of the New Zealand green-lipped mussel (*Perna canaliculus*) for the relief of arthritic symptoms. Evidence of an anti-inflammatory property of the New Zealand green-lipped mussel is believed to have originated in the USA during the screening of marine molluscs for possible anti-tumour activities. A considerable amount of subjective clinical evidence has accumulated suggesting that the preparation may be of benefit in the treatment of arthritic disorders in men and animals. As yet, however, there has been no scientific data to support the belief that it may have anti-inflammatory properties. In the present investigation, however, we believe that it is being demonstrated that, under specific conditions, the material does have a marked anti-inflammatory effect.

This article was written in 1980 and we are now some years further on, during which time the tests have continued. Since then the results of trials conducted all over the world have shown remarkable changes in arthritic conditions when using the green-lipped mussel extract. I will now quote from an article published on research that has taken place at the Victoria Infirmary, Glasgow, the Department of Clinical Pharmacology and the Glasgow Homoeopathic Hospital:

Sixty-six patients took part in the trial. Twenty-eight suffered from classical rheumatoid arthritis and thirty-eight had clinical and radiological evidence of osteoarthritis. All the patients were on the waiting list of the orthopaedic unit of the Victoria Infirmary, Glasgow, for joint surgery. All were taking some form of non-steroidal anti-inflammatory therapy. They were told that they would be taking part in a double-blind trial to assess the value of a new anti-inflammatory preparation, and all were willing to co-operate. Inquiry was made regarding any known allergy to fish or shellfish. The patients were requested

29

to continue all previous therapy unchanged and to take the trial materials as an additional treatment.

*Rheumatoid patients.* The following measures were used to assess the progress of the patients with rheumatoid arthritis: articular index of joint tenderness, morning stiffness, grip strength in each hand, pain as assessed by the visual analogue scale, functional index, and the time taken to walk a measured distance of fifty feet. The patient and the physician also made their own assessments of whether or not there had been an improvement. The patient was considered to have improved when both the patient's and the physician's opinion agreed and there was objective supporting evidence.

*Patients with osteoarthritis.* The progress of the patients with osteoarthritis was assessed by means of the following measures: degree of morning stiffness, pain as assessed by the visual analogue scale, functional index, time taken to walk fifty feet, the range of movements of hip and knee joints, and the patient's and physician's own assessments of improvement. Again, improvement was judged to have occurred when both the patient and the physician agreed that there was objective supporting evidence.

*Conclusion.* This trial suggests that the extract of the green-lipped mussel (*Perna canaliculus*) is an effective supplement or possible alternative to orthodox therapy in the treatment of both rheumatoid arthritis and osteoarthritis. It reduced the amount of pain and stiffness, improved the patient's ability to cope with life, and apparently enhances general health. Added to these benefits is the low incidence of side-effects. It would therefore seem that this substance could be of considerable value to patients suffering from these two chronic and disabling conditions.

A New Zealand dietary expert remarked on the significance of the fact that the green-lipped mussels were eaten raw by the Maoris, as this would ensure that the shellfish would not have suffered any alteration in the nature of the proteins, fats, etc., that they contained. Cooking causes proteins to be denatured and thus they would not have the same beneficial influence on bodily functions as they would when consumed raw. From discussions with tribal chiefs and elders he learned that half of the natural seafood diet of the coastal tribes consisted of green-lipped mussels, while the remaining half comprised seaweeds, crayfish (both cooked), some inshore sea fish and several types of clam. Since this diet has been abandoned the incidence of several diseases and clinical disorders has increased significantly.

In particular, the incidence of rheumatic and arthritic disorders now appears to be the same in the Maori population as in the non-indigenous European population. Many Maoris still seek natural beds of green-lipped mussels to obtain them in the raw state. Others are investing in marine farms to cultivate the mussels themselves. The main purpose of green-lipped mussel cultivation, however, is to produce from them an extract containing all the nutritional qualities. This extract is then freeze-dried (which does not denature the product) and milled to a powder which is then encapsulated in gelatin and marketed.

A further article in the *New Zealand Medical Journal*, this time dated 13 June 1984, reads as follows:

> The results obtained provide strong support for our belief that the extract of green-lipped mussel does indeed contain pharmacologically active material with the characteristics expected of an anti-inflammatory agent inhibiting prostaglandin biosynthesis. Careful examination failed to demonstrate any teratogenic effects which might have explained the results. A possible criticism of our experiments could be that we did not include a study of the

effects of indomethacin or a related drug as a "positive control". These effects have already been observed and, apart from posing logistic problems, the addition of such a group would not have contributed to the interpretation of the results. Indeed, similar studies have not employed such controls either. The present work does conflict with our previous studies which showed that extracts of the green-lipped mussel were only active in suppressing inflammation when given orally. Although the methodologies used in these studies were obviously different, the possibility that prolongation of gestation could be due to mechanisms other than prostaglandin inhibition, and therefore does not imply anti-inflammatory activity, also needs consideration.

One outcome of these experiments has been the establishment of a pharmacological basis for the continued evaluation of the anti-inflammatory activity of the green-lipped mussel. This agent has attracted world-wide attention but has so far lacked laboratory evidence to support its claimed efficacy. Efforts are currently being made to formally identify the active component as a logical extension to the present observations.

Let us consider that it is possible for arthritis sufferers to find temporary relief by way of a painkilling injection or a strong anti-inflammatory agent. However, would that course of action be wise? I have seen patients who had reached the stage when they were happy to subject themselves to a surgical hip-replacement operation — and in most cases this sort of surgery is considered to be very successful. Even some patients who were suffering from advanced joint deterioration have found relief through taking the extract, and among my patients many have been able to avoid such drastic surgery. It is also essential to consider other joints in the body, because arthritis is unlikely to stop at a single limb or joint — it is not selective and doubtless will affect other parts as well. It is a much more complex matter to replace a knee joint than a hip joint and the success rate for the former is much more limited. In this respect I will now quote brief excerpts from an article published in the *Gazette Medicale* 1986, 93, No. 38:

The aim of this study was to evaluate the efficacy of long-term treatment with green-lipped mussel against placebo in arthritis of the knee. The choice of gonarthritis as a model of chronic degenerative arthropathy is justified by the frequency of this arthritic site and the chronic nature and the relative stability of the pain and joint constraint at least in its femoro-tibial manifestation.

Ten clinical criteria were used to assess the efficacy of the tested product. Comparisons between the treated group and placebo group for the consultations following initiation of the trial were done by statistical analysis of each criterion with calculation of averages and analysis of variance with respect to two factors: treatment and time.

The results of the trial indicate an effectiveness expressed by a significant statistical difference between the placebo and treated group in favour of this product for four criteria; the development of three other criteria during the trial stand out equally in favour without the differences reaching statistical significance. Among the original characteristics of the gonarthroses only the severity of functional disability and the radiological stage influence the effectiveness of the tested product which is mainly evident in moderate cases and maximally different at the end of the trial.

Tolerance for green-lipped mussel and placebo was excellent. The results of this preliminary trial support the effective action of green-lipped mussel in subjects suffering from mild arthritis of the knee. They prompt further study of this product on these types of patients to confirm its effectiveness and to determine optimal posology and its mode of action.

The common denominator of most of the above quotes is that there appears to be little doubt as to the anti-inflammatory properties of green-lipped mussel, despite the fact that as yet it has not been possible to identify formally the reason for its therapeutic value. All I can tell you is that it is now a long time since the patient who introduced me to this product was cured. I still see her from time to time and I never fail to be amazed at her remarkable recovery.

# 3

## Dietary Management

*Nau te rourou, naku te rourou, ka ora te tangata.*

*(Your fruitbasket, my fruitbasket, will give life to the people.)*

FROM ALL ACCOUNTS it would appear that the early Maoris followed a healthy lifestyle and had a balanced diet. Not only did they prefer to eat much of their food raw, but even when they had cooked dishes, their cooking methods were such that the food lost only the minimum of nutrients and remained a rich supply of vitamins and minerals. They were particular about isolating raw food from cooked food and certain cooked foods were considered a polluting influence. They were also very hygienic in the preparation of their food. Some of these factors are widely disregarded nowadays, and I am some-

35

times shocked when I see how good food can be abused. Before the European settlers introduced western food to the Maoris, they used to take great care of their diet. This care certainly gave life and strength to the people which was often absent in other indigenous groups and this enhanced the reputation of the Maoris as a stronger and more successful people.

Some of the factors in the preparation of food with which the Maoris were so familiar have been forgotten today. Food is often handled carelessly as many people are more accustomed to eating processed, dried or frozen food than fresh food. We don't think twice about eating irradiated food and do not hesitate to use a microwave oven to put a meal quickly on the table. The early Maoris were exemplary in keeping their food fresh and untainted, and they could certainly teach us a thing or two regarding their respect for food.

I enjoyed hearing the story about the European doctor who was called in to treat one of the Maori chiefs. He took good care of the chief and once, on passing a group of Maori women who were boiling sweet potatoes (I have already mentioned that the kumara is one of the staple foods of the Maoris), he snatched one and the women were shocked and dismayed to see that he touched cooked food with unwashed hands.

Cooking food simply for the sake of softening it was seen by the Maoris as destroying the life within it. If the Maoris decided to cook fish, it was done in the simplest way possible. Thanks to the geysers, the fish was immersed briefly in boiling water, after which it was eaten immediately. Alternatively, they would dig a hole in the soil and would wrap the fish in palm or herbal leaves before cooking it on hot stones. This not only improved the flavour, but also enabled them to enjoy the medicinal benefits of the herbs and plant leaves used.

The Maoris handled their food almost in the manner of a divine ritual and this is surely, as Levi Strauss would say, "a distinction between nature and culture".

It is often thought that the Maoris regarded cooked food as something that belonged to an alien world. The Maoris followed old and traditional rituals for their food preparation. When they displayed the food which had been prepared according to traditional methods, any gathering tended to turn into a feast or celebration. While performing their fascinating dances, for which they are still famous, they would continue to chew their food over and over again, which is something else that we should learn to do nowadays. It seems that we have forgotten that by not chewing our food properly, we make it impossible for the saliva, a natural digestive aid, to mix with it properly, and it is this action of the saliva that causes the food to be digested and absorbed properly.

Not so long ago I heard a professor of rheumatology state categorically that diet had absolutely nothing to do with arthritis. I was sorry that I was not in a position to show him, with the help of some of my patients, how important a good diet is for arthritic sufferers. I am convinced that diet must be considered as one of the most important factors for such patients, because arthritic conditions often thrive on an over-acidic system. One other reason for the arthritis-free society of the Maoris is probably the abundance of the mineral potassium in their diet, which is often a great help for people suffering from arthritic or rheumatic conditions. The sweet potato, or kumara, is rich in this mineral.

No matter what kind of arthritis the patient suffers from, his or her diet must be considered. Without knowing it, many people exist on a sub-nutritional diet and this should be upgraded to an energy-producing diet, which should be especially rich in potassium. Potassium deficiency can lead to rapid calcification in the arteries, muscles and joints. Thus, a diet lacking sufficient potassium causes certain types of arthritis, which are preceded by rheumatic disorders — aching muscles first and stiff joints later. I would advise all people who suffer from arthritis and related diseases to avoid eating any of the following: pork, sausages, bacon, gammon, white flour, white sugar, oranges, grapefruit, lemons, tomatoes, vinegar, mayonnaise, rhubarb, butter, cream and spices.

It is also advisable to reduce the intake of tea and coffee. Salt should be used sparingly and it would be better still to use sea-salt, e.g. Dr Vogel's Herbamare. Rheumatic and arthritic patients should eat plenty of fresh vegetables (either raw or cooked), a salad every day, plenty of fruit (with the exception of citrus fruits), nuts, cottage cheese, honey, brown rice and natural yoghurt. Brown rice is a marvellous source of nutrition, and therefore is of great value for arthritic sufferers. However, the rice must be cooked correctly in order to retain its nutritional value. To keep the life-force in the rice alive, I suggest it is cooked in the following way:


Put the required quantity of rice into a casserole or ovenproof dish. Pour on some boiling milk or, preferably, water. Have the oven preheated to its highest temperature, and place the dish of rice in the oven for ten to fifteen minutes. Switch the oven off and leave the rice inside for five or six hours. When the rice is cooked, chop some vegetables — such as parsley, chicory, celery and cress — and mix them through the rice with a little garlic salt. Before serving, heat the rice through.

I usually advise patients with severe arthritic conditions to adhere to a much more restricted dietary regime. The broad guidelines for such a regime are given below.

*Dietary regime for arthritis patients*

*Preparatory five-day cleaning programme*

Breakfast: fresh or stewed fruit.
Lunch: a salad or vegetable soup; fresh fruit.
Dinner: cooked fresh vegetables and salad; fresh fruit.
Exclude: potatoes, tomatoes, oranges and bananas.
Drink only herbal teas, bottled water or diluted fresh fruit juices.

After five days start on the main diet. A choice can be made from the items listed under each section.

*Breakfast*
Stewed or fresh fruit (excluding oranges).
Cereal, such as muesli or Jordans Original Crunchy Oats sweetened with molasses if necessary, moistened with water, soya milk, apple juice or date juice.
Rye crispbread, brown rice or barley with soy sauce.

*Lunch*
A salad containing any raw vegetables except tomatoes. A celery-based salad is especially good, with grated apple and sprouting seeds added.
Blended vegetable soup or soup from vegetable stock cubes available from health food shops.
Rye crispbread.
Jacket potato.
Any whole grain, such as barley, rice, millet or buckwheat, as long as no polished grains are used.

39

*Dinner*

Fresh sea fish — no more than four times a week.

Shellfish — only twice a week.

Lamb — only once a week.

Pulses such as aduki beans, kidney beans or haricot beans, lentils or chickpeas — no more than three times a week.

Tofu — no more than three times a week.

At least two meals per week should consist of brown rice and sautéd vegetables only.

Cooked vegetables and bean sprouts — only fresh produce should be used.

Potatoes, brown rice, millet, barley or rice.

*Beverages*

China or Earl Grey tea without milk or sugar.

Any fresh fruit juices (except orange juice). Apple juice is especially recommended.

Mineral water.

Herbal teas such as chamomile, juniper-berry or elderflower.

*Seasonings*

Salads may be dressed with Molkosan, olive oil or cider vinegar.

For cooking use olive oil, sunflower oil, soya oil or pure vegetable oil margarines.

Garlic is excellent, but other herbs should be used sparingly. Sea-salt should also be used minimally, as should soy sauce.

For sweetening, honey, molasses or brown sugar may be used.

*Foods to be avoided*

Chocolate, cheese, citrus fruit, beef, pork, poultry, eggs, coffee, red wine, sherry, port, malt vinegar, bread, any flour products (such as cakes, biscuits, buns, pasta, etc.), cordials, fizzy drinks, white sugar, common salt, any processed foods, smoked foods and pickled foods.

*Supplements*
In view of the restrictions in the above diet it is advisable to take certain supplements; for this purpose I usually recommend Dr Vogel's preparations. Take the following supplements daily:

— 2 cod liver oil capsules
— 500 mg calcium pantothenate
— 2,000 mg vitamin C
— 200 IU vitamin E
— 3 vitamin $B_{12}$ capsules
— 4 Kelpasan tablets
To complement the above programme, please use green-lipped mussel extract.

I have been in practice for nearly thirty-five years and during that time I have come to the conclusion that faulty nutrition could well be a causative factor in the development of disease; moreover, I would say that this is more than likely in the case of arthritis. An unbalanced diet can result in an overall deterioration of health and lead to physiological changes in the joints and tissues of the body. A diet which regularly consists of over-processed foods, combined with the toxic influences of meat, tobacco, alcohol, coffee, tea and spices, must at all times be considered a poorly balanced diet.

Back in 1980 the Royal College of Physicians issued a statement requesting that governments and food producers encourage the consumption of foods that are closer to their natural state than the many refined food items that reach the average British table. To my mind

41

there is no doubt that the Maoris remained free from arthritic disease prior to colonisation because of the food they ate and the way they prepared it.

Preparing food correctly is much easier than it may appear at first sight, if only we follow some general rules. The prime factor must be that we should remember what the Maoris did, and learn to respect our food and to know what is good for us. Then, as so many problems are a result of poor digestion, please eat slowly. Saliva, which is essential for good digestion, will be produced plentifully if the food is chewed well. Take time to enjoy your food and so ensure good absorption of the nutrients it contains. Avoid drinking large amounts with meals, as this interferes with the digestion. It is also unwise to eat food that is either very hot or very cold. Remember that, as always, moderation makes sense. Keep food as it is — try not to interfere with it too much or cut it into tiny pieces. Prepare food in such a way that it needs to be chewed well and not just swallowed. Any food that has been roasted will be more difficult to digest. Also remember not to mix vegetables and fruit, as these should never be combined. Avoid the three S's: salt, sugar and stress. Prepare food the Maori way, especially fish; do not overcook it and where possible try to grill rather than roast or fry. Furthermore, I would have to advise against the use of a microwave oven.

The above dietary advice is of great importance when eating for health. Aim for 50–60 per cent of the diet being made up of raw foods, if possible. Remember that an effective dietary programme for rheumatism and arthritis involves increasing its nutritional value. Proper nutrition is a matter of common sense and there is nothing common about common sense! Just remember that a bar of chocolate or a can of fizzy drink has no nutritional value whatsoever and therefore will not help a degenerative condition. We need body builders, not body breakers and proper nutrition is mainly to be found in natural foods and natural remedies. I have plenty of testimonials from patients who have shown that such a regime can be successful. Learn from the Maoris' approach to food preparation. They respected food that had life within it.

Somehow I doubt if our wide choice of tinned, frozen, dried or salted foods provides us with that vitally important life-giving factor. Let us quietly admit to ourselves that such foods are dead in a manner of speaking — they have lost their initial nutritional value while being processed, while raw food retains its vital force within it to repair the wear and tear in our bodies. I have seen many times how a diet high in protein and animal fat can be a causative factor in rheumatic and arthritic conditions.

In answer to your unspoken question as to why I include fish in the diet, I can tell you that fish contains a wealth of essential fatty acids, and it is this factor that is so valuable in staving off arthritic and rheumatic degeneration. Essential fatty acids combined with fish oil give a tremendous boost to the body and in Chapter 5, which focuses on essential fatty acids, I will go into more detail on this.

Another thing that often puzzles patients is the inclusion of tomatoes on the list of foods to be avoided. They point out that the tomato is a popular raw fruit or vegetable, which they expect to be full of goodness. In my dietary recommendations for rheumatism and arthritis I do not actually forbid patients to eat tomatoes, as long as they are fully ripe. A soft tomato may not be as tasty as a firm, crispy tomato, but it is definitely better for our health to eat them ripe and red. This advice is also valid for fruits — only eat ripe fruits. Generally, hard fruits contain too much acid and this is detrimental to arthritis patients, hence the reason why citrus fruits must be avoided completely, in order to keep the citric acid level in the body as low as possible.

Many people also enquire why I advise them to eat dried fruit. Actually figs, dates, prunes, raisins, currants and all other dried fruits are excellent, as long as they are sun-dried and not treated with sulphur. Always be wary of foods that contain any additives or colourings. Dried fruits are rich in potassium which, unless the patient has kidney problems, is excellent for arthritis and rheumatism. You may eat grapes to your heart's content, as well as vegetables such as beans, peas and lentils. These are beneficial because they are high in vegetable protein, which is much better than the protein obtained from meat.

It is interesting to note how much the Maoris used flax. They could not have known why flax-seed oil is so good for rheumatic and arthritic sufferers. The same goes for sunflower oil and sesame seed oil, as these oils are rich in vitamins, minerals and essential fatty acids, which, as I have already pointed out, are good for arthritic conditions.

Let me stress one other aspect of specific importance to arthritis and rheumatism patients — try to avoid constipation at all costs, as this is one of the foremost enemies of people suffering from degenerative diseases. Many diseases originate from a poor bowel function, which explains my insistence on a bowel-cleansing programme prior to patients commencing the advised diet. Waste that is allowed to remain in the bowels tends to ferment and so cause toxicity. Remember the golden rule: in order to avoid problems, whatever is imported should be exported within twenty-four hours.

An ideal start to the day is to eat a bowl of muesli for breakfast with four to six cooked prunes; instead of using milk, mix the prune juice through the muesli. You may like to add half a banana, which will improve the taste and also introduce more potassium. This dish will prove helpful if there is the slightest danger of constipation. The intestines contain billions of different bacteria that aid our digestion and absorption and these bacteria should be given the opportunity to perform their task instead of being allowed to remain idle.

My great friend, the Swiss naturopath Dr Vogel, always states in his lectures that it makes sense to be kind to the friendly bacteria and even if it becomes necessary to fight off the unfriendly bacteria we must be sure to keep the friendly bacteria safe. If this is not done other functions will be affected and possibly destroyed and this would account for the regular occurrence of *Candida albicans*. If harmful bacteria are given the chance to take over, we are likely to experience wind, flatulence and fermentation, and this creates an environment which is conducive to toxicity and impurities, which will eventually poison our bloodstream. For people with sluggish intestines, constipation can be a major problem with far-reaching effects, and we often see how difficult it is for chronically constipated people to eliminate or to get rid of their metabolic waste material.

When I ask if a person is constipated, it is so often denied, and yet when I ask how often a motion is passed, the answer is always in a multiple of days rather than hours. Just think of babies, who have a bowel movement virtually after every meal, and this is often the case with animals as well. For adults it would be ideal to evacuate the bowels mornings and evenings and a good intestinal balance can only be reached by eating the right foods.

To encourage better bowel movement you may opt to fast occasionally. Alternatively, you may prefer to use a laxative such as Linoforce from Dr Vogel, which is an excellent natural laxative containing flax-seed and senna as its two main ingredients.

A change of air or water could well bring on a temporary period of constipation and if this happens while travelling or on holiday, eat at least one portion of natural yoghurt daily, as this encourages the bacteria to function properly. The acid/alkaline balance is extremely important for our well-being and this in turn depends on the protein/carbohydrate balance, which may require some alteration when suffering from constipation. To put it to you in layman's terms: carbohydrates burn like wood in a fire and we know that if we burn wood, we are left with only dust and ashes in the grate. Yet if we burn coal on the fire we can expect to find cinders and slag among the ashes. The body is like a fire. If we supply it with good fuel, the burning process will be clean. For good fuel now substitute good carbohydrates, by which I do not mean white sugar or white flour. Carbohydrates from a reliable source will burn up cleanly and will leave the body easily. High-protein food, however, is like coal, and leaves behind undesirable waste in the body. Living on a diet rich in animal protein is like feeding the fire with coal, as it is difficult to digest and equally difficult to eliminate.

My grandmother was a great believer in castor oil and recognised it has a cleansing effect and will encourage bowel movements. Most meat-eaters suffer from constipation as animal protein is difficult to digest and absorb; the same is true of dairy products, which constitute the highest source of saturated fat in our diet.

During the Second World War I was only a youngster and although I was not aware of it at the time, despite the general shortage of food, people were actually healthier than they are today. Certainly in the Netherlands, which was an occupied country, food was in very short supply and many people suffered as a result; nevertheless, the incidence of degenerative diseases was actually lower than today. Sometimes my mother tells me about the problems the Dutch people were faced with and she claims that they possessed much more courage and inner strength despite, or because of, the little there was to eat. The food that was available was nutritious. Meat was certainly in desperately short supply, as was cream, while we had forgotten the taste of chocolate. We considered ourselves lucky to have some greens from the fields and occasionally we managed to catch some fish from the river, which turned our meal into a feast. Yet the population's general health did not reflect this lack of food.

The lesson we should learn from this, therefore, is to be careful with meat, particularly pork. More than any other kind of meat, pork is extremely high in animal fats and animal acids, which are detrimental to our health. It is better to eat poultry or game; in chicken the fat is found between the muscles and over the surface and in game it is right under the skin. With regard to poultry, chicken is the wisest choice, as duck and goose are relatively high in saturated fats and cholesterol.

Remember that you are a living creature and as such you require food that contains life within it. The life-force within us will help our immune system to stand up to all the attacks on our health which we have to face daily. Too many chemically produced foods can be harmful as their nutritional value will have been largely destroyed and by eating them we would be inviting illness and disease.

Why do we consider it necessary to interfere so much with nature? Why is it that we have spoilt our food and our drinking water and the God-given air we breathe? We should return to nature and for confirmation of this we only have to look at the Maori dietary habits and we will see that before colonisation they suffered very little illness or disease because their immune systems were much stronger than they are today.

The Maoris regarded food almost as a divine gift, and what a tremendous encouragement it must be to see food as a gift from God which should be loved and respected. Learning about the care and appreciation that the Maoris lavished on their food, the sensible precautions they took and how they handled food, we see a sharp contrast with the picture today, when it is common practice to abuse this gift of nature in all kinds of ways. Our bodies are unique, highly intricate machines which can easily be damaged or destroyed by supplying the wrong fuel. Thus, it is always a small miracle when ill-health and disease are overcome by the introduction of a well-balanced diet.

I cannot understand doctors and rheumatologists who attach no value to diet because I have seen at first hand what a wholesome diet can achieve. The results cannot be disputed as they speak for themselves and I myself have treated many patients who have been meticulous with their diet and have proved the point that in the treatment of a degenerative condition, diet can be a decisive factor.

I wonder whether the Maoris instinctively understood the principle behind the familiar saying "All healing comes from within and the body heals itself". Many people think that if they eat plenty of meat and eggs and drink plenty of milk they are doing the right thing. Well, they are wrong! Especially for arthritic patients, this is a complete misconception. Remember that a change of diet often results in changes in the body and a change for the good is likely to stimulate the body into applying its healing powers in order to restore itself to health.

Were you to decide to bring about some changes in your diet and substitute certain foods with more nutritious ones, you would certainly be rewarded with an improved feeling of well-being. The following old Maori saying is further proof of their perception:

*Hi kahi, hi kahi — Some food, for some food.*

# 4

## Vitamins, Minerals and Trace Elements

THE DIET OF the early Maoris was varied and of such a quality that it provided an ample supply of vitamins, minerals and trace elements. On the whole it can be said that they did not suffer from dietary deficiencies because their choice of food was well balanced. Nowadays this is no longer the case and, like other people, the Maoris have also had to introduce vitamin supplements to their diet, as their deficiencies have become obvious. Sadly, it is the same all over the world: it has become necessary to supplement the diet with additional vitamins, minerals and trace elements, as too often these vital ingredients are lacking. Whilst a balanced diet is essential for everyone, this is particularly true of arthritis sufferers.

Of course, not just any food supplement will do. Every arthritic patient must be assessed on an individual basis and his or her specific requirements worked out accordingly. However, for the purpose of this book, I will give some advice of a more general nature.

It is staggering to realise that in Britain alone, more than five million people suffer from one or other form of arthritis. I heard these figures confirmed by rheumatologists speaking on a recent radio programme. Most of us are confused about the various different types of arthritic conditions. However, to put things in perspective, we only need to ask ourselves how many people we know with arthritic complaints of one kind or another and then we will realise the scale of the problem.

The biggest fear of many of the people who come to my clinic for help is that they will become permanently disabled because of their problem. Thankfully, I can reassure most of them that this need not be the case. The majority of people whose arthritis is in its early stages can lead a normal life and will be able to control their condition by paying heed to some of the advice given in this book.

Few people are fully aware of the tremendous number of different kinds of arthritic conditions, but for obvious reasons I will concentrate here on the more widely known ones.

Osteoarthritis is a degenerative condition of the joints from which millions of people suffer, even though they may not always be aware of it. Often the pain, discomfort, or even stiffness they experience is accredited to circumstantial conditions, such as an injury, while many a time its true cause is the onset of arthritic degeneration.

Another major arthritic condition is rheumatoid arthritis. The symptoms are quite different to those of osteoarthritis and its treatment requires a totally different approach. How comforting it is to know that the green-lipped mussel extract is suitable for the treatment of all kinds of arthritis, especially when taken as part

51

of a programme of supplementary vitamins, minerals and trace elements. Green-lipped mussel, when included in such a programme, is often referred to as a food supplement, and because of present-day farming practices, such supplements are often essential as the nutritional value of food is lower than it used to be.

Unfortunately, juvenile arthritis (which, as the name suggests, predominantly affects the younger generation) has become much more common in recent years and this also is largely a result of dietary deficiencies. Thank goodness, with the right treatment and the patient's co-operation, this condition can definitely be brought under control and more often than not it can actually be cured. However, it must be understood that this is totally dependent on the willingness of the patient to co-operate.

It is quite a different matter in the case of joint degeneration, or wear and tear, which is mostly beyond a cure. Even so, there is tremendous hope for the average arthritis sufferer, as the pain and discomfort can certainly be relieved. Bearing this in mind, we must explore further the need for supplementary vitamins, minerals and trace elements.

Everyone needs a regular supply of vitamins and generally these are obtained from food. If we eat fresh vegetables and fruit on a regular basis we can be sure that under normal circumstances we will ingest sufficient vitamins. Where necessary, this intake can be supplemented with vitamin preparations and occasionally this course of action is essential. I will try and explain why this is so.

A great deal depends on how we treat our food. Looking back to the chapter on the dietary management of the early Maoris, we learned that they prepared and cooked their food correctly, something which appears to be proving more and more difficult nowadays. When vegetables are overcooked most of the vitamins will be lost because they disappear down the sink when the cooking water is poured away. It is similar with a carton of orange juice: once opened, the vitamins will soon disappear. Therefore fruit and vegetables should be eaten as fresh as possible. There is no harm in occasionally using frozen or tinned foods, because modern conservation methods are so advanced that it is now possible to retain many of the vitamins in the food. In fact, it is often during the defrosting process that the greatest loss of vitamins takes place.

Certain types of vitamin are destroyed more easily than others, and this is particularly the case for vitamins B and C, as these are water-soluble. For this reason, please take care when rinsing or blanching vegetables or fruit.

Patients often ask me how they can tell if their vitamin intake is adequate. It is, of course, possible to find out by doing blood tests. However, even if the vitamin supply has been deficient for some time, the symptoms will not be such that they would indicate serious illness. Complaints such as lack of appetite, listlessness, lack of concentration and sleeping problems, may all be experienced. If these complaints do not sound familiar and a sensible diet is being followed, it is fair to assume that the vitamin intake is adequate.

Another question I am frequently asked is if it is possible or dangerous to take too many vitamins. In general, it can be said that water-soluble vitamins such as vitamin C and the B vitamins, which are important for rheumatism and arthritis, can cause only minimal damage — even if the recommended daily intake were to be exceeded one-hundred fold. All surplus intake will be eliminated from the body by way of the bladder.

Fat-soluble vitamins, such as vitamins A and D, have a much smaller safety margin. Vitamin A does not represent any danger until the recommended daily intake is exceeded by up to ten times the suggested amount. The safety margin for vitamin D is five times the recommended daily dose.

Vitamin C plays an important role in the control and treatment of rheumatism and arthritis. It is true that vitamin C not only cures colds, but is capable of much more. It is also a very important anti-oxidant, and helps to sustain and rebuild the immune system. We need to understand that the human body is incapable of manufacturing most vitamins. The exceptions to this rule are vitamin D and niacin (vitamin $B_3$), and even these are produced only in minute quantities, so that a supplementary intake, either through food or specific vitamin preparations, is usually necessary.

Rheumatic patients, especially, often have a greater need for vitamins as a result of their regular use of medication. The use of certain medicines can alter the rate at which the body absorbs, uses, stores and eliminates vitamins. Such medication includes certain antibiotics, diuretics, oral contraceptives, tranquillisers and pain-killers.

Vitamins enable us to convert food into energy. It is therefore impossible to actually improve one's medical condition simply by taking vitamins. When feeling listless it is, of course, a different matter, because then a course of vitamins will no doubt boost the body's energy production.

As most vitamins deteriorate when food is heated and when exposed to oxygen, they can rapidly disappear from our food. Incorrect food preparation and a monotonous diet both contribute to a lack of vitamins in our diet, in which case it is sensible to make up for this deficiency with a vitamin supplement.

Alcohol and tobacco users should be aware that vitamins break down more quickly in their bodies, resulting in a greater need for supplementary vitamins. Physical exertion also speeds up the metabolism and so increases the body's need for vitamins and minerals. Older people, whose bowels may function less efficiently, are often less capable of absorbing the required vitamins and minerals from their food. Another group of people who may experience problems are those who have difficulty in masticating their food because of ill-fitting dentures. All these factors are significant when deciding whether or not to take supplementary vitamin preparations.

Over the years the metabolism appears to slow down and the body requires less energy. The appetite frequently wanes and as a result the diet deteriorates. Problems may then occur in the body as a result of a specific vitamin deficiency, or because of continued use of medication, or simply as a result of natural changes in the metabolism. Vitamins C, D (or extra sunlight) and the B complex will invariably be helpful in such circumstances.

It is not an old wives' tale that when the letter 'R' appears in the name of the month a vitamin supplement may be required. In years gone by, cod liver oil and vitamin C were taken on a regular basis during the winter months. Lower temperatures demand extra energy from the body and the greater contrast between the indoor and outdoor temperatures places added strain on the immune system. During the winter, fresh vegetables are often grown in greenhouses without the benefit of as much sun as summer vegetables receive; as a consequence these vegetables contain less vitamins.

Numerous vitamin preparations are available that will help us to sustain our vitamin levels during the winter months, the best known of which are vitamin C, multivitamins and cod liver oil capsules. In addition to these, vitamin E, spirulina, calcium, garlic and wheatgerm oil can also be beneficial.

It may be helpful to include here some specific groups of people who appear to be especially susceptible to vitamin deficiencies, and for whom it is therefore recommended to use vitamin supplements, especially if they suffer from rheumatism or arthritis.

A good intake of vitamin A is essential for people who suffer from arthritic conditions. Vitamin A is a nutrient obtained from liver, fish oils and dark-green leafy vegetables. It is used by the thymus gland — the key organ of the immune system — and it also helps to strengthen our barriers against the outside world. It is important for the maintenance of the mucous membranes found in the lungs, the throat, the nose and the mouth, which form a sticky trap for particles and micro-organisms. It also helps cells in all parts of the body to grow and repair themselves. Vitamin A's affinity with cells means that it is needed by all parts of the body. It plays a part in the formation of blood and, where cell turnover is at its greatest, the bones and teeth.

Certain forms of vitamin A have different characteristics which in nature appear at various stages of conversion and metabolism. Vitamin A is often taken in combination with vitamin D, which is vital for the proper absorption of calcium, and phosphorous, which is needed to build healthy bones and teeth. A good supply of vitamin D, sometimes known as the "sunshine vitamin", is essential for arthritis sufferers.

This is also the case with vitamin B. It is often necessary to take a vitamin B complex preparation because these vitamins cannot be stored in the body. Processed foods will have lost their vitamin B content, and the body's ability to absorb these vitamins is also affected by our sugar intake. At times of great stress the balance of bacteria in our intestines can be disturbed, reducing the availability of vitamin B for use by the body. Vitamin B usually occurs in a complex form in nature. The B vitamins all seem to work together so it is important to take a B complex preparation. The major role of the B vitamins is to keep the nerves and nervous system in order, including the brain. They also assist in releasing energy from carbohydrates, helping the metabolism of proteins, maintaining the muscles of our digestive tract — which are used for repair — regenerating the liver and maintaining healthy eyes, skin and mucous membranes.

Now I will say a little more about vitamin C. It is essential that arthritis and rheumatism sufferers take additional vitamin C. It is needed all over the body, from our brain to our connective tissues. Without vitamin C our natural immunity would crumble since it goes into action at skin level as well as in the bloodstream. Vitamin C is involved either directly or indirectly in every biochemical process that takes place in the body. Because it is needed everywhere, some experts suggest that we need enough to keep ourselves saturated and I have often prescribed vitamin C in large quantities for arthritic sufferers. As it is a vitamin that we, unlike most other forms of life, can no longer synthesise, we have to obtain it on a daily basis from our food. Yet cooking or storing food incorrectly will immediately result in the loss of vitamin C.

We need additional vitamin C when we are faced with demanding situations, as it is essential for the effective function of the hormonal adrenal system. It is used to maintain the immune system and to repair tissue. Iron, which is also often deficient in arthritic patients, is absorbed better with vitamin C, while the absorption of certain other nutrients, such as selenium and vitamins A and E, is completely dependent on an adequate vitamin C supply. Vitamin C is an excellent anti-oxidant. It helps to protect nutrients and fatty acids and, in particular, it prevents over-reaction when oxygen is involved. One of the reasons why arthritis and rheumatism sufferers must supplement their intake of vitamin C is that they are often prescribed large doses of aspirin, antibiotics and other drugs, which deplete the vitamin C resources obtained from the diet. This is one lesson that has been learned as a result of research programmes and the technology is available to prove its importance.

Vitamin E — alpha tocopherol — is another valuable anti-oxidant, and is the body's most powerful ally in helping the defence system, or natural immunity. It is the prime agent that prevents the fatty acids from reacting with oxygen to form harmful toxins known as lipid peroxidites. Not only does vitamin E protect fats in the body, but it also protects other vital nutrients such as vitamin A, the B complex vitamins, and vitamin C. The anti-oxidant vitamin E allows the more efficient use of oxygen by the blood and muscles, so it is favoured by sports people who are working to increase their stamina and endurance by training their heart and circulatory systems.

A safe supplementary vitamin programme is as follows:

| | | |
|---|---|---|
| Vitamin A | — 2,500 iu | — 1-2 times daily |
| Vitamin B complex | — 100 mg | — 1-3 times daily |
| Vitamin C | — 1,000 mg | — 1-2 times daily |
| Vitamin D | — 400 units | — 1-2 times daily |
| Vitamin E | — 400 units | — 1-2 times daily |

This is a safe combination, which can possibly be increased, but only under guidance of a medical practitioner. I have worked for years with Nature's Best vitamins in the treatment of arthritis and rheumatism, and I trust their products completely.

After lengthy research I have developed a formula called Imuno-strength, which has the specific purpose of strengthening the immune system, as the name implies. Not only does Imuno-strength contain the necessary vitamins but, as an extra aid, such plants as echinacea, devil's claw and ginseng have been added. For hundreds of years these have been used to support the body's natural defence mechanisms. Imuno-strength has combined tradition with science, and the result is a supplement designed to support our natural defences by ensuring proper nutrition.

A well-functioning immune system is undeniably essential in our efforts to remain healthy. It is a natural, but also very complex, system involving both mind and body, which today is being faced with more and more challenges, as we have to adapt to this fast-moving, ever-changing world where the risks of degenerative disease appear to be growing continuously. The carefully chosen ingredients of Imuno-strength will be of great benefit to the natural defence system and the formula is a combination of the following:

| | |
|---|---|
| Vitamin A | —900 mcg (3,000 iu) |
| Riboflavin (vitamin B) | -- 10 mg |
| Vitamin $B_6$ | — 50 mg |
| Folic acid | — 50 mcg |
| Pantothenic acid | — 50 mg |
| Vitamin C | —165 mg |
| Vitamin E | — 80 iu |
| Calcium | — 19 mg |
| Iron | — 1 mg |
| Magnesium | — 3 mg |
| Manganese | — 50 mcg |
| Selenium | —100 mcg |
| Zinc | — 20 mg |

| | |
|---|---|
| Devil's claw | — 100 mg |
| *Echinacea purpurea* | — 200 mg |
| Ginseng | — 15 mg |

Although there is much confusion about the use of vitamins, minerals and trace elements, we only have to realise that common sense tells us that nature demands a little extra help every now and then. As far back as 1922, two scientists, called Evans and Bishop, noted that something present in lettuce prevented fatal resorptions by animals which had been fed a rancid diet. The unknown substance was Vitamin E, which permitted an animal to have offspring. Evans called this substance tocopherol, from the Greek words *tokos*, meaning "childbirth" and *phero*, meaning "to bring forth".

During the period 1922–24, Mattill and his collaborators were engaged in investigating this new substance. Research into vitamin E is still continuing, but all I can say is that I would be lost without it. In cases of blood circulatory problems and as an anti-oxidant (as a means of protecting the tissues) vitamin E plays an important role.

Again, if we look at the work of Linus, Pauling and Cameron on vitamin C, we find ourselves wondering what would we do without it today! Every vitamin is important in its own way and guidelines are necessary to help the public to understand the intricate workings of the immune system.

Vitamin F is one of the less well-known vitamins. It is an essential fatty acid and is significant because the body is incapable of its production. In Chapter 5, which deals specifically with essential fatty acids, I will come back to this substance, which is of crucial importance in the treatment of arthritis and rheumatism.

Minerals and trace elements are of equal importance to our health. As biologically active components of the earth's crust, minerals are not synthesised in the body — they have to be obtained from our food. However, the soil in which our crops are grown and on which our animals are grazing is becoming depleted of its mineral content. Calcium, iron, iodine, zinc and selenium are all minerals that are in danger of becoming in short supply; I have even heard farmers complain that a cow or a calf has died because of a lack of certain minerals, which means that the soil in that pasture is lacking these minerals. In Scotland this often happens because of the tremendous rainfall, which washes away some of the minerals in the grass.

Minerals affect the absorption of vitamins and work with them in the body. They are also vital components in many of the chemical catalysts called enzymes, without which life itself is unsustainable. Minerals demonstrate their importance to us in obvious ways. Iron enables the blood to transport oxygen. Calcium is used to construct the bones and teeth. Zinc is found in prostatic fluid, and selenium, potassium and sodium help work the pump that breathes life into individual cells.

The scientific and medical authorities have confirmed the fact that the human body is composed of minerals. The foundations of the earth and the human body are both dependent on salt. Salt itself is recognised as the basis of all physical life. In the human body twelve different colours of salt can be found. The water or moisture passing through the different colours of salt creates twelve different acids. Other acids are created by two or more coming into contact with each other as they flow through different organs of the body. This, from a scientific standpoint, proves the alkaline and acid theory to be more or less correct.

From day to day, the mineral level in the human body fluctuates as we perform our daily tasks. The circulation of the blood must be efficient if it is to eliminate these dead or decomposed minerals in order that the body may attract new substances. If the circulation and elimination are insufficient, then the body degenerates and becomes diseased. This must be clear to every thinking person. Some wonderful results have been achieved in the treatment of degenerative diseases with the help of minerals; thus, as we are concerned with arthritis and rheumatism, we must certainly consider some of these substances in greater detail.

First, let us consider iron, particularly as so many arthritic patients also display symptoms of anaemia. Iron is available in many foods, but sometimes we need to use a supplement. Alfavena — a Bioforce product with alfalfa as its major ingredient — has proved to be of great benefit because of its natural iron content. I have often prescribed this when extra iron has been needed because of a serious deficiency.

Urticalcin — another Bioforce product — is a combination of calcium and nettles, and is ideal for patients who need help to rebuild their muscles and tissue and transport the mineral iron throughout the entire body. When I use the term "muscles", I wonder if you are aware how extensive is the network of muscles and fibrous tissue that covers the whole of the body. There are even muscles that are connected to the cartilage in the joints of our body. Whenever the flesh connects with this so-called elastic fibre, it acts as a muscle. We have muscles from the top of our head all the way down to our toes. We have scalp muscles and muscles that move forwards and backwards. Remember that bones never move on their own — it is the muscle that moves the bone. Even the involuntary nervous system should be included here, as muscles become impaired and must be treated. Muscular fibre connects with the lymphatic system, then again with the arteries and so we can go on.

This explains why it is so important that the muscles are adequately nourished. The mineral iron provides strength for all these different muscles. It is not only iron — all minerals are important for their individual properties and they all interrelate.

Now for a brief look at calcium. This mineral is responsible for building the bones and teeth and is essential for the balanced function of the nerves and muscles. It is also of importance in blood clotting and is considered essential for the maintenance of normal levels of cholesterol in the blood. It tones the elasticity of the muscles, including those relating to the heart. Calcium has an association with amino-acids, with hormone production and its function is also closely linked with magnesium.

There are seventy-two minerals and trace elements present in the body, and a good balance in the majority of these must be maintained to assist in relieving the condition of rheumatic and arthritic people. If there is a deficiency of minerals in general, it must be rectified.

A balance of calcium and magnesium is particularly important for the health of muscles and bones. Magnesium, which is found in potatoes, vegetables, bananas, seeds, nuts and rice, can sometimes be lacking when the individual does not have a balanced diet. In this case the dietary intake can be supplemented with Magnesium Plus — another product from Nature's Best. Magnesium is of importance for the growth of bone tissue and for an efficient calcium metabolism. It also helps the reproduction of cells and energy.

Now for a look at phosphorous, a mineral which also helps the growth of strong bones, as well as combating tiredness and muscle weakness. Again, maintaining a good balance of phosphorous with calcium is important. Good sources of phosphorous are beans, nuts, lecithin, eggs and fish.

I also often prescribe a zinc supplement as there is generally a deficiency of zinc in the soil. Zinc plays a very important role in growth, tissue repair and the immune system and is therefore essential when dealing with degenerative diseases. It has been claimed that in today's refined and processed foods, 80 per cent of their natural zinc content can be lost, which is why a zinc supplement is necessary in many cases. The Maoris, of course, had an enormous zinc intake, because shellfish and other seafood accounted for such a large part of their diet, and the good health they enjoyed serves as an excellent example of the value of this mineral.

One of the minerals that is given considerable coverage in the press for arthritic and rheumatic complaints is selenium. I cannot help thinking that the media sometimes exaggerate their claims of newly discovered remedies for certain conditions. A specific substance may be hailed as a panacea for a specific illness or ailment, then one or two months later that same substance may be slated as useless or, even worse, harmful. Self-help is all very well, but often the sensible thing to do is to consult your medical practitioner if you are considering introducing a new substance into your programme. Many of the claims made for selenium are indeed very impressive, and many of my patients have benefited from this product.

The results obtained from some recent trials are fascinating. It appears that a staggering 79 per cent of the people involved reported to have noticed an improvement in their condition and some actually claimed that the improvement was noticeable from as early as one week after starting a course of selenium. In these trials, selenium was taken alongside vitamins A, C and E and the results were overwhelming. At the end of a three-month trial, 2,000 questionnaires were returned, representing 67 per cent of the total who had been asked to participate, and the response was most optimistic.

The mineral selenium is essential for our health, although it is needed only in minute quantities, and I am delighted with the outcome of the trials. Our soil is supposed to have a certain selenium content but, as with zinc, it is becoming very sparse. Hence the frequent need to supplement this mineral in other ways.

Let us not forget the importance of potassium, which acts as a secondary agent of cellular breakdown in the acid/alkaline system, affecting the joints. Potassium is essential for health and it can be found in potatoes, bananas, dried fruit, molasses, cider vinegar and apricots. It is known to alleviate the impaired function of the neuromuscular system. Because of its properties it is suitable for use in the treatment of allergic conditions. Remember, however, to take care when introducing supplementary potassium to the diet if the patient has a history of kidney problems. Nature's Best has brought out a very interesting remedy — Natural Iron with Blackstrap Molasses. This syrupy nutrient, which is a by-product of the process of refining sugar, provides us with the ideal base on which to promote the absorption of iron gluconate and is also very valuable because of its potassium content.

Copper is not normally considered as a mineral, but supplementary zinc promotes the level of copper in the body, which is essential to enable the conversion of iron into a state in which it can be absorbed by the blood. The metabolism also requires a combined copper and zinc input, although the ratio is 25 mg of zinc to 1 mg of copper. Copper is important in it own right for the production of healthy red blood cells and it plays an integral part in the functions of those vital enzymes I have already mentioned. Copper will stimulate enzyme production and effectiveness, and should therefore be introduced into the programme for arthritic conditions.

I would understand if by now you are slightly dazed by the list of vitamins and minerals I have just outlined to you. So any of the substances mentioned would greatly benefit one's health, but it is ridiculous to suggest that you should visit your health-food store with the intention of purchasing all the supplements mentioned. Well, the good news is that Nature's Best has done all the hard work for you and have designed a mineral supplement to give you choice and flexibility, called Chelating Mineral Complex. Two tablets of this remedy will provide you with the following:

| Calcium (from oyster shells) and calcium phosphate | — 750 mg |
| Magnesium (as oxide) | — 375 mg |
| Phosphorous (as calcium phosphate) | — 186 mg |
| Potassium (as gluconate) | — 42 mg |
| Iron (as fumerate) | — 20 mg |
| Sulphur | — 6 mg |
| Iodine (from kelp) | — 0.15 mg |
| Zinc (as gluconate) | — 142 mcg |
| Manganese (as gluconate) | — 94 mcg |
| Copper (as gluconate) | — 52 mcg |
| Chromium (as orotate) | — 15 mcg |
| Selenium (as seleno-methionine) | — 10 mcg |

Molybdenum (as potassium molybdate)   —   5 mcg
21 amino acid mix                         —400 mg

This combination will give you all the recommended minerals in one fell swoop and has been designed to make life easier, while still enabling you to benefit from the supplementary minerals.

Before concluding this chapter I would like to say a little about pantothenic acid. This is part of the vitamin B complex and is water-soluble. It occurs in all living cells and is widely distributed in yeasts, bacteria and the individual cells of animals and plants. Pantothenic acid is synthesised in the body by the bacterial flora of the intestines. It stimulates the adrenal glands and increases the production of cortisone and other adrenal hormones — which are important for healthy skin and nerves — and as such it plays a vital role in cellular metabolism. It participates in the release of energy from carbohydrates, fats and proteins, and in the utilisation of other vitamins, especially riboflavin. Pantothenic acid can improve the body's ability to withstand stressful conditions. An adequate intake of pantothenic acid also reduces the toxic effects of many antibiotics.

The richest sources of pantothenic acid are liver, egg yolks, wholegrain cereals, royal jelly, soya beans, dried peas and brewer's yeast. Because of all its medical properties it is highly recommended for arthritic patients and this is one of the reasons why I advocate the regular inclusion of brown rice in their diet. If a balanced diet is followed, deficiencies are unusual.

Some time ago I read an exclusive interview with Dr Christian Barnard in a Dutch magazine, in which he stated that he had treated himself successfully for arthritis. He pointed out that he had geared his whole diet to providing an over-abundance of pantothenic acid.

BY APPOINTMENT ONLY

Taking into account the information contained in this chapter, the Maori diet must have been even more remarkable. It seems incredible that their food intake was balanced to such an extent that it contained all the essential vital minerals and trace elements to keep them healthy and fit and, moreover, free from rheumatism and arthritis.

# 5

## *Essential Fatty Acids*

FATTY ACIDS, KNOWN collectively as vitamin F, or EFAs, are fat-soluble. Unsaturated fatty acids usually come in the form of liquid vegetable oils, while saturated fatty acids are usually found in solid animal fat. Saturated fatty acids are metabolised by the body more slowly than unsaturated fatty acids.

The body cannot manufacture the essential unsaturated fatty acids and they must be obtained from food. Wheatgerm, seeds, golden vegetable oil, and cod liver oil are some of the best sources of essential fatty acids. They are important for respiration, and facilitate the transportation of oxygen by the bloodstream to all cells, tissues and organs. They also help to maintain resilience, or immunity, and lubrication in all cells and combine with protein and cholesterol to form membranes that hold the body cells together.

Vitamin F helps to regulate blood coagulation and

performs a vital function in breaking up cholesterol deposited on arterial walls. It is essential for normal glandular activity, especially the adrenal glands and the thyroid gland. It nourishes the skin cells and is essential for healthy mucous membranes and nerves.

The unsaturated fatty acids function in the body by co-operating with vitamin D in making calcium available to the tissues, assisting in the assimilation of phosphorous, and stimulating the conversion of carotene into vitamin A. Fatty acids are needed for the normal function of the reproductive system.

The stomach, small intestine and pancreas normally produce liberal amounts of fat-splitting digestive enzymes necessary for the conversion of fats into fatty acids and glycerols (broken down fatty acids). The latter are absorbed through the walls of the intestinal tract and are then transported to the liver, where they are usually metabolised as a source of energy. These changes must take place before the nutrients can enter the blood, if food allergies are to be avoided.

The digested fat is taken from the gastro-intestinal tract as fatty acids and glycerol. These then enter fat-collecting ducts that finally carry the fat to the lymphatic system, which is primarily concerned with collecting body fluids and returning them to the general circulatory system. The fatty acids are stored in the adipose (i.e. containing massive amounts of fat cells) tissues.

Absorption of fat is decreased when there is increased movement in the gastro-intestinal tract, and when there is an absence of bile to break it down. X-ray treatments and radiation destroy the essential fatty acids within the body, although their destruction can be prevented if large doses of vitamin E are taken. Vitamin F is easily destroyed when exposed to air.

There is often a little confusion concerning the use of oils which contain essential fatty acids, but any criticism regarding the use of these oils is unfounded. Fish has always been used as a food source. Through the ages people have also used vegetable oils or oils from seeds and herbs. Certainly, the Maoris' diet was rich in essential fatty acids, with fish being an important source of nutrients.

Only recently I read that shark liver oil is now under investigation as a dietary supplement. Unfortunately, the media have sensationalised this discovery and suddenly everyone's expectations are raised. Let us not fool ourselves into thinking that a new product is being launched, because from Maori history we learn that shark oil was used regularly for internal and external purposes. The oil was used in their rituals, where it served a symbolic purpose, and in some of their legends we can read about confrontations with sharks, eventually ending in glorious victories, with the shark supplying the meat for their tribal feasts.

Today the shark is known to be remarkable in the animal kingdom, in that it does not suffer from cancer. This knowledge could be the reason why the use of shark liver oil, in combination with green-lipped mussel, is recommended for degenerative disorders such as osteo and rheumatoid arthritis, psoriasis and even cancer.

From the examination of a shark's skeleton certain conclusions can be drawn about its apparent immunity to cancer. It is believed that protein in the shark's cartilaginous skeleton contains a substance that strongly inhibits the growth of new blood vessels in tumours, thereby restricting tumour growth. Shark liver oil is also a powerful non-toxic anti-inflammatory agent. I doubt very much whether the Maoris were aware that the use

71

of both green-lipped mussels and shark meat provided them with a combined angiogenesis-inhibiting property, giving them — as it were — a layer of immunity in the joints. Such inflammations are often found in the cartilaginous joints of people with osteo and rheumatoid arthritis.

Researchers agree that the primary anti-inflammation component in shark cartilage is a family of complex carbohydrates, called mucopolysaccharides. Two members of this family, A and C, are often used in nutritional medicine to control inflammation. Because shark liver oil contains these specific carbohydrates, it is thought to be highly effective for anti-inflammatory purposes. Moreover, sharks have powerful immune systems. From their omnivorous lifestyle as scavengers, it is clear that they are able to successfully combat bacteria and viruses and also certain chemicals which would kill a human being. Inflammatory disorders are often associated with immune dysfunction and the immune-modulating substance works to provide a synergistic effect.

In tests with rheumatoid and osteoarthritis patients, shark liver oil has been shown to be useful. The data obtained indicates significant improvements in cases of injury or stiffness of joints and muscles.

In previous studies of the Eskimo dietary habits it was very clearly shown that using fish oils can reduce the risk of heart attacks. Indeed, many studies have clearly shown the benefits of including fish in the diet. In my own research into multiple sclerosis I have made sure that these dietary studies have also been included and applied. The studies on Eskimo dietary habits concluded that the very low incidence of heart problems, cancer and arthritic complaints in Eskimos could most likely be attributed to the properties of fish oils.

I was one of the first practitioners in Great Britain to use oil of evening primrose, having recognised the need for essential fatty acids. When I started to prescribe this food supplement, which is a rich source of essential fatty acids, I was ridiculed by the medical establishment. Today, I am delighted to see that the National Health Service also recognises the importance of essential fatty acids in the treatment of osteo and rheumatoid arthritis as part of a complex programme.

Essential fatty acids as dietary factors present in the evening primrose were initially isolated in 1929 by researchers at the University of Minnesota. The dietary importance of the seeds of this little plant, with its bright yellow flowers, was also known to the South American Indians. Some of our own poets have even written odes to this small, but attractive, plant. Since that time its beneficial effects on healing seem to have been largely forgotten, until they were rediscovered during research at the University of Minnesota. It proved to be very complex establishing exactly why this extract is beneficial, but it has been concluded that one very important component, gamma linolenic acid, or GLA as it is often referred to, is essential to health. Particularly when combined with a fish oil, it has been proven to be of great benefit to countless people.

For many people who have difficulty in converting linolenic acid into GLA, oil of evening primrose has proved its value, providing people with health benefits which they did not previously possess. The most important of these is the conversion of linolenic acid into GLA. Until GLA is produced it cannot be turned into the fatty acids which are vital to the health. Linolenic acid is a polyunsaturate

73

and one of the most important substances in our food. This essential fatty acid, like vitamins, is necessary for the maintenance of a healthy body. Scientists have now reached the conclusion that linolenic acid plays a significant role in the prevention of all kinds of degenerative illnesses as well as heart disease.

In this day and age there are many reasons why people become deficient in GLA. Convenience foods, hard margarines, and products which are high in saturated fats such as butter, milk and red meat, can hinder the production of GLA in some individuals. It is also an accepted fact that serious illness, including cancer, can be caused by over-indulging in alcohol. This creates a deficiency in certain elements, which in turn causes the body to stop producing GLA.

Oil of evening primrose is one of the richest sources of this nutrient. Earlier in this book I mentioned prostaglandins. This group of substances was initially identified in 1935 when it was thought to originate in the prostate gland, as the name implies. The vital action of prostaglandin E is very important in cases of rheumatism and arthritis and the Delta-6 — desaturated enzyme — is of great importance with regard to EFA, since it converts to GLA in the diet, the precursor of prostaglandin A. This provides yet another reason to use green-lipped mussel, together with a combination of evening primrose and fish oil.

Investigations have shown that during the processing of vegetable oils the EFA enzyme can be inhibited. There are two types of essential fatty acids, namely the Omega-3 series, found mainly in marine fish oils, and the Omega-6 series, mainly of vegetable origin. Both series are incorporated into cell membranes and both are precursors of the eicosanoid biosynthesis. The eicosapentaenoic acid

— EPA — of the Omega-3 series of EFAs has attracted a great deal of interest over the years in connection with the well-publicised health and fitness of the Eskimo communities. Many studies in predominantly fish-eating communities have also found that the incidence of heart disease, arthritis, rheumatism and psoriasis is much lower than average. Little attention has been paid to the Maoris in recent years because their change of diet has been so extensive.

The potential of the Omega-6 fatty acid, namely gamma linolenic acid or GLA, has been widely investigated in clinical trials relating to a wide range of medical disorders. In Scotland, research conducted under the guidance of Dr Iain Cloughley has shown that marine fish oil together with oil of evening primrose has been of benefit to many patients. Dr Cloughley has remarked on the irony that our modern hi-tech medical establishments are only now beginning to accept the claims of folk remedies, because the supposed benefits of marine fish oil and oil of evening primrose have been dismissed for generations as old wives' tales.

Let us now look more closely at some of Dr Cloughley's reports.

### Specification of evening primrose
Specially selected seed oil rich in polyunsaturated essential fatty acids occurring in the natural triglyceride form. The oil contains the important Omega-6 series fatty acid GLA and also linolenic acid and has been extracted under the most exacting quality control requirements.

### Specification of Marine 18
Specially selected and purified fish oil prepared exclusively from cold-water Atlantic species. The oil is a rich

source of essential fatty acids, especially the Omega-3 fatty acids EPA and DHA (docosahexaenoic acid). The polyunsaturates are in the bio-active cis-form and occur as natural triglycerides. An important feature of this oil is the very low level of cholesterol.

### Specification of Marine 25
Specially selected and purified marine fish oil unusually rich in the important Omega-3 polyunsaturated fatty acid EPA. This natural triglyceride oil also contains high levels of DHA, another important essential fatty acid. All poly-unsaturates are in the bio-active cis-form.

### Specification of Omega combination
A 50/50 blend of Marine 25 fish oil and evening prim-rose oil giving a rich, natural triglyceride oil contain-ing both the Omega-3 and Omega-6 series essential fatty acids.

Below each of these specifications Dr Cloughley pro-vides a long list of the individual fatty acids contained in the individual products mentioned, which I consider to be too technical to be of any real interest to the non-scientific reader.

I find it ironic when I think back to the times when I was ridiculed for my determination to prescribe remedies containing these oils for my patients. For exactly the same reasons that I insisted on prescribing them, they are now available on prescription in more than thirty coun-tries. These remedies are used as nutritional supplements because of their richness in essential fatty acids and I am happy to see that these old and tried methods are making a comeback and are now widely acknowledged as being beneficial to people's health. The safety of GLA and EPA as nutritional supplements has been tested since the early 1970s, both in Britain and abroad, without any indication of side-effects.

Scientific researchers foresaw that in some circumstances a considerable advantage would be gained from GLA supplied directly to the body and the constituents of the oil, and their beneficial effects, must have influenced the good health of the early Maoris. Not only are these benefits obtained from the seeds of the evening primrose, but it is now known that blackcurrant and borage seeds contain similar properties, and this discovery is especially interesting because the Maoris also used borage seeds. Today, however, it is important to use these products carefully and only cold-pressed oil of the highest quality is recommended for use for the purposes under discussion. I find it fascinating that thirteen medical schools in Britain are presently involved in the research studies in this field and it has already been established that a high potency is sometimes necessary.

Evening primrose oil is thought to be an important ingredient that is metabolised by chemical messengers or hormone-like substances, which control different metabolic pathways. Human breast milk is one of the best known sources of correctly balanced EPA and GLA and experts have been trying to find a more convenient source. To date, the evening primrose plant is still one of the richest known sources of GLA, from which the body produces vital prostaglandins, and its oil has now become a standard GLA supplement. Nature's Best already provides some excellent products and I am currently involved in formulating certain remedies containing combinations of oils to help alleviate specific conditions.

The amazing oil of garlic — *Allium sativum* — is also currently the subject of extensive research. Although garlic capsules and tablets have been used for quite some time now, oil of garlic is also considered extremely useful for rheumatic conditions. Garlic oil is rich in vitamins B, C and D, as well as zinc, copper, sulphur, and crotonic aldehyde. This last constituent plays an active role in destroying harmful bacteria, which are often one of the underlying causes of rheumatism and arthritis, and also delays degeneration and the ageing process.

Boericke, in the ninth edition of the *Materia Medica,* notes that the blood temperature drops 30–45 minutes after taking a substantial dose of garlic oil and also that fat deposits in the body are greatly reduced. Although garlic oil is an old remedy and one that has been largely forgotten in recent times, its importance should not be underestimated.

The same applies to cod liver oil, which I like to see taken in combination with oil of evening primrose. The Dale Alexander cod liver oil treatment is held in high esteem by many, but let me warn you that unless this remedy is taken as part of a complex programme, it will be only moderately successful. Such a programme should also include a well-balanced diet, as described in my earlier book *Arthritis, Rheumatism and Psoriasis.* It should also include a course of vitamins, minerals and trace elements, as well as green-lipped mussel, together with some herbal remedies. For this purpose I often prescribe Imperarthritica, a Bioforce remedy made up of herbs, essential fatty acids and cod liver oil.

The Chinese maintain that the condition of the skin is a useful indicator of deficiencies in the body. From the skin it is certainly possible to ascertain a lack of essential oils, and we often see that dry skin is common in arthritic patients. With this in mind, I will now quote, with his permission, some instructions given by my good friend Leonard J. Allan, DO, which he published in a series entitled *Diseases of a Modern Age*:

Dry skin is a big problem today. Bigger than you probably realise. I'd say that one out of every two people has dry skin in one form or another. Today, people of all ages — teenagers, children, even infants — are suffering from some form of dry skin. Wherever I travel, I am continually amazed at how many people are affected.

Dry skin and arthritis are just two sides of the same coin. Many arthritic victims have dry, flaky skin. And many people with dry skin eventually go on to develop arthritis. When your body is dry, it's dry all over — whether it is the skin, the joints or anywhere else.

To correct dry skin you have got to get your body to produce its own moisture — from the inside.

This programme is built around an easy-to-live-with, all-round, wholesome diet that emphasises fresh vegetables, salads, fruits, whole-grains. It includes unsalted butter, eggs, fish, such as salmon, halibut and mackerel, cod liver oil and oil of evening primrose.

These last four foods — unsalted butter, eggs, fish and cod liver oil — contain the four best oils for your skin. As you may know, cod liver oil tops the list.

Now we come to the second half of the diet — the foods to avoid — junk foods, refined products, and sugary foods and liquids. The diet also excludes inferior-type oils and fats such as margarine, fried foods, potato chips, roasted nuts, and so forth. These oils will only clog the skin instead of nourishing it.

Cod liver oil can do for skin in six months what diet alone would take five years to accomplish.

Cod liver oil has an almost magical ability to lubricate the skin. I can't explain it; I don't fully understand it, and yet I've seen it time and time again. Perhaps the best explanation I can think of is that cod liver oil is a marine oil. It doesn't come from the land, as other oils do.

It comes from the oceans — the richest area of nutrients known to man.

Be sure to drink your liquids ten minutes before a meal or three hours afterwards.

The timing of your liquid intake is critical to your assimilation of oils. You should drink water, tea, coffee, alcoholic beverages or other "oil-free" liquids at least ten minutes before meals. If not, then wait until three hours after meals.

If you drink liquids with meals — as most people do — as little as 5 per cent of your dietary oils will reach your skin to lubricate it. That is a pitiful amount. It explains why your skin can dry out in the midst of plenty.

However, when you drink liquids at the proper times, as much as 50 per cent of the dietary oils will reach the skin. That is ten times the oil absorption. Quite an amazing difference.

*List of liquids which you should avoid:*
1. Regular tea and coffee.
2. Frozen, fresh or bottled fruit juices.
3. Soft drinks.
4. Acetic acid vinegars.
5. Powdered imitation drinks.

The Dale Alexander cod liver oil programme is often misunderstood and for that purpose I will now give you the correct instructions, which must be followed carefully:

1. To achieve the best results, take your cod liver oil mini-milkshake one hour before breakfast. If more convenient, you may drink the mixture just before bedtime — at least four hours after your evening meal (or last food).

2. It is important to use a 4–5-ounce screw-top jar. If you use a larger jar, more of the oil will be left clinging

80

to the inside surface of the jar, and your body will receive a lesser amount.

3. To mix and emulsify the cod liver oil with whole milk is a simple procedure. Pour two ounces of whole milk into a screw-top jar. The jar should be large enough to hold four to five ounces of liquid.

4. Add one tablespoon of cod liver oil. Shake vigorously for about fifteen seconds. The cod liver oil mini-milkshake will then become foamy. Drink the mixture immediately.

5. Do not take any food after this oil mixture for at least an hour.

6. If you are allergic to milk, or do not like it, you may use two ounces of freshly strained orange juice to prepare the mixture.
*Note: Cod liver oil is much more effective and works faster when it is mixed with milk.*

7. Cod liver oil capsules are not to be substituted. The content of the capsules is quickly captured by the liver, since gelatin promotes digestion, and the skin linings are denied proper lubrication.

8. After a while, you can start to reduce the frequency of the mini-milkshake. When you see that the dryness of your hair or scalp has been corrected, or when a normal supply of wax returns to your ears, then you can begin to ease up on your cod liver oil intake.

9. Do not stop taking the cod liver oil mini-milkshake suddenly. At first, consume the mixture every other morning, instead of daily. Continue to follow this plan for approximately six months. Then, the use of the oil can be reduced to once a week.

*Note*
If you have a troublesome gallbladder, or have had it removed, use only one teaspoon of cod liver oil in the mixture and take it on alternate days.

Other people who should deviate from the above rules are those suffering from ailments like high blood pressure, heart disease and diabetes. These individuals may not assimilate oils very quickly. They should take the cod liver oil every other night, or just twice a week.

People with eczema, psoriasis, dermatitis, any type of ulcer, or a skin irritation characterised by nerve involvement, should use only *whole milk* to mix their cod liver oil. People suffering from these ailments are often allergic to the citric acid and fruit sugar of the orange.

Again, we have seen that the Maoris, although they may have done so unconsciously, lived a healthy lifestyle and avoided arthritis because they used oils which contained essential fatty acids. How clever they were in using flax-seed oil with fish oils! In one of their stories I read about an occasion when some Maoris caught seventy snappers, which were carefully placed in a watertight vessel. These live fish were subsequently used for one of their big feasts. From the book, *Legends of the Maoris*, we learn that in the days before the white men came, the Maori ceremonies involving fish were steeped in ritualistic tradition. The white men have a lot to answer for, because they were the initial cause of the great changes that have taken place in the Maori diet. Modern science is all very well, but one should never overlook the lessons that can be learned from historical folklore. These lessons have withstood the test of centuries, and the results cannot be disputed.

# 6

## Herbal Medicines

ACCORDING TO MAORI FOLKLORE, minor illnesses and diseases were treated with herbal or vegetable remedies and their knowledge in this field was really quite remarkable. It is a great pity that so much of this knowledge has subsequently been lost and it is only because some of those methods were recorded by early settlers that we have any idea of the Maoris' extensive medical knowledge.

We have already heard that the Maoris were fastidious in the preparation of their food and that many foods would be wrapped in leaves prior to being cooked. These leaves would serve a dual purpose: not only were they medicinal, but they also improved the taste. The food would be eaten together with the leaves that had been used in its preparation.

One of the favourite leaves for this purpose was the mountain celery pine. We now know that these leaves have great diuretic properties and are therefore excellent for cleansing the kidneys. They also used the leaves of the cabbage tree, and these kept them safe from inflammation and helped to retain flexibility in their muscles. I was impressed to learn that as well as using the bark and leaves of many trees, the Maoris were also familiar with a variety of seeds. They used these as medicines and for their tribal rituals. Indeed, without their knowing it, the Maori diet of leaves, bark and seeds, was probably extremely beneficial in the prevention of conditions such as arthritis and rheumatism.

Nowadays, flax-seed oil is gaining in popularity because of its richness in essential fatty acids. Centuries ago the Maoris used the flax-bush for many purposes. They wore flax cloaks, made from flax fibres woven into a coarse linen fabric. They also extracted oil from the seeds of the flax-bush, and used the heart-leaves, and even the flower. It appears that they attributed specific powers to the leaves of the flax-bush, as these were supposed to enable them to find and win their true love. The central leaf of a flax-bush would be modelled into the shape of a canoe, in which a pebble was placed representing the person who was going to send it on its way. This symbolic vessel would then be launched on the waters of the lake. A gentle wind was supposed to carry it to the girl of the sender's dreams and direct her thoughts towards him. While the flax-leaf canoe was floating away it was customary to sing a song, pledging love and devotion. Songs and dances, chants and incantations were the very life of the Maoris and song was very much the natural expression of these warm-hearted people.

I was impressed to learn that the Maoris were aware of the mistletoe's medical properties. Mistletoe — *Viscum album* — was widely used by the Maoris for the prevention of illness and disease and nowadays it once again holds an important place in herbal medicine. Since the rediscovery of this plant it has been used as an excellent remedy for balancing blood pressure, to treat migraines and epilepsy, and is also used by cancer patients. Mistletoe is a semi-parasite that requires a tree for its "host" and the unusual characteristics of this plant have earned it a well-deserved place in herbal medicine. Judging by the extent of the Maoris' knowledge of herbal medicine, they must have been very observant: the large number of herbs used by the Maoris that have been largely forgotten by the West is truly astonishing.

There exist many legends about mistletoe in many countries, but it seems to me that the Maoris knew so much about this plant simply through observation. The Maoris say that the berries of the mistletoe are the tears of the plant, which cause us to reconsider and repent and remind us of life in general. They also say that the mistletoe is a life-and-death plant. Consider the fact that it attaches itself to a host tree and then grows like a parasite, in much the same way as a cancer develops. In this way mistletoe reminds us of its medicinal purposes. It is a very strange plant, because, unlike any other parasite, it has green leaves. It does not grow upwards either, but downwards or sideways instead. Unusually, it flowers in the autumn and produces berries in the spring. It is indeed one of the oldest remedies for the prevention and sometimes cure of disease, and realising this helps us to understand why the modern school of Rudolf Steiner has earmarked it as a very powerful remedy.

The myths and legends of the Maoris provide us with an insight into their thought processes: the things they liked or disliked, the things they valued or hated. This insight gives us a certain understanding of their appreciation of the natural medicinal properties and other characteristics of plants, flowers, leaves, seeds and roots.

Herbal medicine was bestowed on mankind for healing and we must realise that we are dealing with living objects with an identity of their own. The ancient knowledge of herbs forms the backbone of modern medicine. We must not view herbal medicine from a pharmaceutical point of view; it is not always possible to give a pharmaceutical explanation for the effects of a plant. They must be regarded as something very special. Today's scientists cannot comprehend that all living things — human, animal or vegetable — have an extra dimension. I believe that plants have a soul of kinds, and we have to look a little deeper than at the action of the plant. We must, in fact, view it holistically, as we should, for example, view our bodies. Every herb has a message. We may try to capture one particular aspect or component and manufacture a synthetic remedy, but if we take the wider view, as the Maoris did, and take into account all the healing properties, we will receive the message loud and clear that herbs were given to us for healing.

Reading up on the Maori traditions has reminded me of the time I spent in China. There, it is believed that all illness is disharmony. To be specific, disharmony in mind, body and soul. Universal methods of healing are plentiful and in the Chinese Pharmacopoeia — dating back to 2700 BC — we can read about herbs that were used successfully for healing purposes in those days, while only recently have we in the West become acquainted with some of these remedies.

We must learn to look at the characteristics of plants in the same way as the old masters of herbal medicine did. They tried to read the signs by studying the way the plant developed, and this information was interpreted into herbal compositions for the treatment of specific illnesses.

Some time ago I visited the archaeological excavations of an old monastery in the Scottish Borders and then a few months ago I read an article about some of the finds at this site. The following article appeared in the archaeology section of the *Sunday Observer* of 16 September 1990:

Dr Brian Moffat, whose speciality is archaeological "dirt", is uncovering the secrets of one of Britain's most important medieval hospitals. Searching for clues among the ancient hospital's rubbish, he has already discovered important new evidence of the medical remedies used by the monks at the Hospital of the Holy Trinity in Soutra, Scotland.

"Most archaeologists are obsessed with craft objects and will lovingly clean a piece of pottery. But at Soutra it is the so-called dirt clinging to the pottery which can tell us much about how the Augustinian monks cured the sick," he said.

Soutra, seventeen miles south-east of Edinburgh on the edge of the bleak Lammermuir Hills, has been bypassed by the modern world. "Most medieval hospitals were in what are still existing towns. Although Soutra was once on the main road from Scotland to England, the route was changed and it now lies beneath barley fields," said Dr Moffat. "The archaeological remains are therefore well preserved and readily accessible."

Thanks to the co-operation of the local farmer, Dr Moffat and his team have been excavating Soutra for five years. Financial backing for the work has come from dozens of organisations, including the Pharmaceutical Society of Great Britain, the Royal Colleges of Surgeons and Physicians in Edinburgh and the National Museums of Scotland.

Among the typical finds at Soutra is a fourteenth-century ointment jar, which still has traces of grease inside. An analysis of the grease reveals that it was made with forty-two separate ingredients, including flax, myrrh and balsam. This "cocktail" of herbs suggests that the preparation may have been polypharmaceutical, a deliberately complicated concoction made to disguise a secret preparation to prevent it being copied.

Blood dumps have also been found, preserved in deposits of clay. Documentary evidence from the Middle Ages reveals that blood-letting was widely practised by monks in order to quell their "sensual desires". It is believed that they took enough blood to lose consciousness, probably about three pints, up to once a month.

The substantial quantities of blood found in Soutra's clay appears to confirm this practice. The samples are now being investigated by the Scottish National Blood Transfusion Service, which is hoping to be able to analyse blood type and illness present.

Dr Moffat is also excited by his investigations into the hospital's drains. "We have found deposits of quicklime. It has been assumed that it was not until the late eighteenth century that quicklime's use as a disinfectant was discovered. But its presence at Soutra suggests that the monks may have known about its properties in medieval times," he said.

The Hospital of the Holy Trinity, which was well established by the twelfth century, treated everyone from beggars to kings. Its most illustrious patient was Edward I, who was at Soutra during three military campaigns. The hospital finally closed in 1562.

"It will take at least another five years to finish the excavation and even longer to analyse the material," said Dr Moffat. "Our findings are throwing important new light on medieval medicine and may even have relevance to medical treatment in our own times."

I found this article fascinating reading and I fully agree with Dr Moffat when he says that some of the conclusions we have drawn from his findings may well be relevant to medical treatment today. It certainly shows that centuries back our forebears had their own specialised knowledge about herbal medicine and it should not surprise us that the Maoris knew so much, even though their knowledge would have been different, as the flora of New Zealand is obviously very different to ours in the West.

Universally, we see that in earlier centuries "medicine" was in fact herbal and, until the nineteenth century, illness was mainly treated with herbal and natural medicines. It seems that around that time the medical establishment was not too happy unless a herb could be re-worked into a drug with clearly defined pharmacological action. This was certainly the case with digitalis, although initially it caused major concern that the whole of the plant was not used, which would probably have saved some of the early victims' lives, when this drug was tested.

It seems that lately the import of herbal products is valued at a figure in excess of US $100,000,000 a year in the United States alone, and there is little doubt that phytotherapy methods are well received all over the world.

Great understanding and knowledge shines through the expression accredited to the seventeenth-century British botanist, Robert Tradescant, who said that God has given us plants, herbs and flowers as hieroglyphics to show us their medicinal purpose. The scientific theory is often seriously considered by scientists with some botanical knowledge. It is interesting that the Italian Gianbattista della Parta (1538–60) recognised a similarity between the helio or scorpio herb, and a scorpion. In olden days great value was attached to the personality and characteristics of the plant, and today we must be careful not to overlook this. Medicine should look back to its roots.

Despite the fact that we now live in a nuclear age, the message and efficiency of the old herbal remedies still emphasises the point that we are born in, and belong to, nature. We ought to rethink and study afresh the unknown secrets of herbs and move ahead according to the principle that the secrets of nature will be unfolded to enable us to help people meet the demands of life. We must adapt our way of thinking in order to make sure that recently discovered scientific facts do not erase the knowledge that has been gained over many centuries.

Cartesian logic shows that the characteristics of a mixture are likely to be quite different to the sum of the characteristics of individual parts. We see this clearly with the artichoke, which has beneficial effects on the liver. By using the whole of the artichoke, the benefits to the liver have proved to be quicker and more effective than if a single component of the artichoke were used. The combination of traditional and modern science has resulted in renewed acceptance of phytotherapy. This word is a combination of the Greek words *phyto* meaning "plant", and *therapeia* meaning "curative". In phytotherapy it is taught that when the whole of the plant is used, possible side-effects are often neutralised by other components of that same plant.

To the Maoris, phytotherapy and hydrotherapy were a natural way of life. For hydrotherapeutical purposes they would use water from the sea, lakes, geysers, or hot springs, whichever was readily available. They did have preferences and certainly the hot springs were the most beneficial for rheumatic complaints. In about 1865, Father Mahoney, a Roman Catholic priest who was crippled with rheumatism, heard of the healing waters of Te Pupunitanga. He walked slowly and painfully along the native tracks until he came to the medicinal spring and camped beside it. After a week of bathing in its healing waters, he was completely cured. Such was the fame of this cure that the spring has since been known as the Priest's Bath.

It was typical of the Maoris that they gave names to all their springs and many were very descriptive. The sulphurous waters still have great medicinal powers. Before universal pollution became a sad fact of life, sea-water was well balanced and it was the source of life to millions of fish. The Maoris, living close to nature, must have instinctively realised the importance of such balance, whether it be in the water or in their food. Yet that balance was lost when modern food was introduced. For thousands of years the plants, the geysers and the hot springs were the only means of treatment for the Maoris. It was the same for many other civilisations throughout the world. Today, by allowing certain influences to become established, we have become vulnerable to many self-inflicted diseases.

Many of the herbs used by the Maoris can be found in the present Heath and Heather range. Their remedy for rheumatic pains has similar ingredients to Maori herbal mixtures. Many remedies are designed for the purposes of alleviating pain, but with rheumatic patients in particular, constipation is a major problem that must be dealt with. There is a large variety of laxatives available, a few of which have linseed as the principal ingredient. We should remember that it is very important for rheumatic patients to pass a motion every day. This motion must not be forced and preferably it should take place at set times, so that the patient can be sure that there are no problems in that direction.

Many people nowadays enjoy a cup of herbal tea. Not everyone drinks it for medical reasons, but often because they enjoy the taste. Dr Vogel's kidney or golden grass tea is a blend of many herbs and this combination is an excellent kidney cleanser. Garlic capsules are often recommended as part of this cleansing programme. Nettle tea has become increasingly popular recently, and this popularity can be largely attributed to a newspaper article about a lady who lost her balance and fell into a bed of nettles while gardening. Her initial discomfort can easily be imagined, but after twenty-four hours she suddenly realised that the arthritic pains she normally experienced had disappeared. This was due to the active ingredients in the nettles.

Many plants have active ingredients which do not cause side-effects. Some of their medicinal effects we have learned about from medical folklore and others have been stumbled upon by accident. The nettle is an effective painkiller and will help the metabolism and anaemia, while it also has an important regulating action. If we were to go out to pick berries it would be useful to know that some of them have pain-relieving qualities too. Chewing a few of these berries each day will help to relieve pain.

As we have seen, the Maoris had a great liking for potatoes, in their case the sweet potato, and fresh potato juice is highly recommended for arthritic people. Without peeling the potato, wash it well, then grate it and extract the juice from the pulp. Only a little juice will be obtained but this should be drunk first thing in the morning, immediately after it has been prepared. This is an excellent remedy with which to filter the acid in the stomach.

Patients with all types of arthritis have been successfully treated with the green-lipped mussel extract together with Dr Vogel's Imperarthritica. These two remedies complement each other for most forms of arthritis. Sometimes I feel it is also necessary to prescribe a kelp supplement, as this sea plant helps to absorb a great deal of toxicity in the body of a rheumatic person. Kelpasan, like Imperarthritica, is a Bioforce remedy and the ingredients of both are listed below:

*Imperarthritica*

| | |
|---|---|
| *Polygonum aviculare* | — knotgrass |
| *Solidago virgaurea* | — golden rod |
| *Petasites officinalis* | — butterbur |
| *Potentilla anserina* | — silverweed |
| *Achillea moschata* | — yarrow |
| *Betula alba e folium* | — white birch and leaves |
| *Viscum album* | — mistletoe |
| *Equisetum arvense* | — horsetail |
| *Colchicum autumnale* | — meadow saffron |
| *Mentha piperita* | — peppermint |

*Kelpasan*

Kelpasan is made of pure algae from the Pacific Ocean with all the trace elements. It is a natural supplement for iodine deficiency and a prophylaxis for goitre. It stimulates cell metabolism in the endocrine glands, and increases mental and physical capacity.

As many rheumatic patients can be anaemic it is often advisable to take Alfavena, which is also a Bioforce preparation. The contents of this remedy are as follows:

*Alfavena*

| | |
|---|---|
| *Extr. Medicaginis* | — alfalfa extract |
| *Trit. Urtica* | — stinging nettle trituration |
| *Extr. Avena sativa* | — oat seed extract |

It is always rewarding to hear how well a patient has reacted to a specific programme, especially if that patient lives far away and it is unlikely that I will see him or her again. Many of the letters I receive are an expression of happiness and delight at the success of the prescribed treatment. An American lady, who had consulted me during a holiday in Britain, wrote:

"I am cured of all the pain in my back and legs, and I felt easier within hours after taking your remedies. I cannot express in words my astonishment at getting rid of these pains so quickly and efficiently, while I have suffered them for so long. Since the course of treatment has been completed, I have not suffered a recurrence of those familiar pains."

I cannot deny that it is gratifying to receive such letters, but I hasten to add that rheumatic or arthritic people should not think that their symptoms will clear up over night. Nevertheless, it is marvellous to see that often the pain can be reduced.

Another patient I particularly remember was a lady who suffered from quite severe kidney and liver problems. These problems are sometimes a side-effect of rheumatic conditions, and are caused by changes in the level of acidity in the body. She wrote to tell me of her delight at the immediate improvement she experienced and wanted me to know that she thanked me from the bottom of her heart. The average programme for the treatment of arthritis generally consists of some herbal remedies, occasionally combined with a preparation of essential fatty acids. In cases of constipation, castor oil compresses are recommended, and the results are usually speedy and satisfactory. The lady with the additional problems in her kidneys and liver was advised to use green-lipped mussel, Imperarthritica, Alfavena, vitamin C and compresses of warm castor oil. These compresses are especially good for supporting the kidneys and the liver. They should be used for three consecutive days or, in special cases, for five consecutive days. For the benefit of those who may wish to try this simple remedy, I have provided some guidelines below.

*Directions on the use of warm castor oil compresses*

*Requirements*
Clean white flannelette or white cotton material (e.g. old sheet)
Castor oil
A wide shallow pot
A plastic sheet to cover the mattress
A strip of plastic to cover the area to be treated
White towels
White swab/facecloth or hand towel
Hot water bottles
Blanket
Bicarbonate of soda (1 teaspoonful)
Warm water (1 pint)

*Method*
Cover the bed or mattress with a plastic sheet and a towel. Cut the flannelette into a strip long enough to wrap around the body and wide enough to be folded into three layers to cover the organs to be treated. Gently warm the castor oil and immerse the flannel in the pot. The compress should be saturated, but not dripping. Place the warm compress over the area to be treated and cover with the strip of plastic; then cover the plastic with a white towel. Place the hot water bottle(s) over the area under treatment and cover the patient with a blanket to keep warm.

The compress should be left in place for a minimum of forty-five minutes (or longer if desired). After removing the compress, wash the area down with a swab or facecloth soaked in a mixture of warm water and bicarbonate of soda.

Understandably, patients are often impatient and want to know how long it will be before they will recover, or at least experience some improvement. One can never tell; the body has the last word. There are often several stages of recovery. First, the limbs may loosen up, the energy increases, and the digestion may improve considerably. Then there may be a stage when the patient experiences a deterioration in his or her condition. This is the time when many patients are inclined to give up hope. I can assure you that this stage is only temporary and must stress that the programme should be continued. When the joints feel more painful, it is only a sign that something is happening within the body. The patient may remain in this stage for some time before reaching the next stage.

The third stage can be compared to a process of rebuilding the muscular tissue and will result in greater freedom of movement. Exercise will become easier before the fourth stage is entered — when it is very encouraging to see a patient making a true recovery. It is fantastic to witness people's reactions at this stage, when they know that their perseverance has been worthwhile. There will have been times when all the effort seemed in vain and it would have been tempting to forget all about the programme of treatment. But always remember: "without battle, there is no victory".

At all times the patient must be encouraged to fight on. After all, if we look at life in general, we realise that it is comparable to a chemical process; moreover, we know very little more than our ancestors did. People with degenerative diseases should be aware that life is the constant renewal of cell tissue. If life is indeed a chemical process, then degenerative disease is a relentless breakdown of cells. So we cannot afford to live with this unrealistic idea that symptoms can be treated with chemical drugs. It is time to realise that we cannot expect complete healing unless the cells are encouraged to renew themselves.

When I take a step back and look at mankind in a slightly more detached way, I can see that it is hemmed in by so many influences and that no real effort has been made to gain control of the impulses that run loose in the world. It has been, and still is, easier to let things go on as they are rather than exert the will required to redirect certain forces. We are all creations of emotions, passions and circumstances. What the mind will be, what the heart will be, what the body will be, are the desires that are shaped according to the drift of life. We take too many things for granted. If we take one glance at the great kingdom of herbs, it should become immediately obvious that these were given to mankind for healing purposes.

If we just look at what it means to function on full energy, enabling us to do our day's work and enjoy the beauties of nature, we will be surprised to find how much of our life to date has been adrift. How little have we done to find out about how that power operates!

Just look at the life of any living thing and consider the effort of self-expression. The tree directs its branches upwards towards the sunlight and its roots downwards in search of water. We call this inanimate life, yet it represents a force that comes from the source and is directed to some equilibrium. Man is a higher form of life than that of other animals, and animal life is higher than that of vegetation. We all have millions of tissue cells in our body — more than our mind can conceive or our pencil could write in figures. Yet none of these cells originated other than in a plant, nor could they have originated other than in some force that existed in or of the cell itself.

Consider for a moment the tremendous energy, sometimes called bio-energy, that exists in herbs and vegetables of any kind. To call it a force would be more precise than energy, and yet we do not require a scientific name, because its existence is a basic fact. Actually, whenever a new scientific book is written, the author believes that his invention of a few thousand technical words may well establish a new science and draw all students to their feet. He is inclined to load the volume with impossible terms, until the reader's interest sinks with its weight. Once in a while a short simple word is required to explain a new idea, but the disposition of scientific writers to invent long technical terms has loaded their specialist literature with an oppressive burden that for the most part strangles its meaning.

There is no place on this globe without energy. The air is loaded with energy and the friction caused by different temperatures meeting can create alarming electrical conditions. Water is a liquid union of gases and is charged with electrical, mechanical and chemical energies, any one of which is capable of doing service, or great damage, to man. Even ice in its coldest phase has energy, for it cannot be subdued. Its force has been known to break mountain rocks into fragments.

The innate energy of man is so great that we have barely scraped the surface. If we look at life in general, then we can be grateful that wherever we go there is a lesson to be learned, and that lesson is often of great value if only we are prepared to acknowledge it. Sometimes it hurts, sometimes it brings joy, but if we look at it objectively, we will have many reasons to be grateful.

While writing on the subject of herbs, I remember the winter of 1944–5. As a child, while the war was raging, I could not understand the death and destruction that surrounded us. That is when I came to the conclusion that the creator of mankind must have created a herb for every ill and every disease. I am grateful that circumstances have steered my life towards investigating the great wonders of nature.

During the war, through underground connections, my mother was asked to help at a nursing home near Arnhem. While my mother was working I was looked after by an elderly monk, who lived in a monastery next to the nursing home. He became my greatest friend. The herb gardens surrounding the monastery were most impressive, but what was more important an influence was what he taught me about the energy and force in nature which was present in herbs and other plants. This old friend taught me, as young as I was, some of their medicinal applications. Today, having been in practice for many years, I still thank God daily for His wonderful gifts and the opportunities I have had to learn about them. One of these opportunities has been to learn about the ways of the New Zealand Maoris and I have endeavoured to use this knowledge for the benefit of my patients.

# 7

## *Water Treatments*

WATER PLAYED A large part in the day-to-day lives of the Maoris. Of course, it was a major source of their food and as such they depended on it. I imagine that it must have been impossible to live in New Zealand, with its abundance of springs, waterfalls and lakes, without being affected by water. Many of the Maori legends mention the discovery of lakes, pools or waterfalls and all these were named according to the circumstances in which they were discovered. We have already read about Hinemoa swimming across the lake to join her beloved, and I have also specifically mentioned Father Mahoney bathing in the health-giving water of a spring, ever since referred to as the Priest's Bath. These are only two occasions, but almost all of the Maori legends seem to relate to water in one way or another.

I have read that it was not unusual for a teacher to pour water into his pupils' ears. It was believed that this would open up the ears so that the pupils might hear their lessons more clearly, and so enhance their learning capacity.

However, while water was used for such superstitious rituals, it was also considered as a cleansing agent. It was thought that water could rid people of certain unpopular characteristics and it could rinse away minor misdemeanours. A sprinkling of water was supposed to remove any bad habits and render the person clean and revitalised. This indicates that water was used for symbolic purposes and it was in that sense, as well as for their physical needs, that water was respected by the Maoris.

Living water was an intrinsic part of the lives of the Maoris and it was thought to restore life, to rejuvenate and to give people better health. Hot mineral springs are found in great numbers in New Zealand. Some of these springs are characterised by considerable thermal activity and the majority of them have a curative effect on people's physical ailments. Hot springs sweep over the beach between the low and high watermarks. By low tide it is possible to take a pleasant natural hot bath at a very comfortable temperature. For arthritic sufferers the effects of bathing in these springs, which are so rich in minerals, can sometimes be astonishing.

In the centre of the northern island a number of active volcanoes are to be found and it is said that the valley of geysers provides a supply of energy so rich that it surpasses even the electrical energy supply from the national grid. The minerals in these areas are unique and it seems astonishing that such a relatively small area of approximately 100,000 square miles contains such a wealth of natural powers and minerals.

In the ocean surrounding New Zealand extensive areas of submarine plateaus rise from the deep levels of the

Pacific Ocean to the South Tasman Sea. Sea-bathing and swimming were common practice for the Maoris and formed an intrinsic part of their health regime, as they needed to remain fit to fight their many battles.

The area surrounding the Rotorua township is dotted with hot springs and geysers and is famous for its thermal activity. The region is known as Whaka, which is a shortened version of its official name of Whakarewarewa. At one time this was a famous settlement and it was the township that later gave its name to the surrounding area of geysers, boiling pools of water and mud. These thermal pools have become renowned for their tremendous healing powers. Bathing in mud pools and the effervescent water of the geysers is widely reputed to protect one from rheumatism and arthritis. I have advised patients who have been travelling to this part of the world to visit the thermal pools as often as they could.

On the basis of this, I maintain that arthritic people are able to enhance the effectiveness of their treatment programme with water therapies, even if the water used does not contain the minerals present in the New Zealand waters. There is nothing to stop people taking a sauna or a steam bath, or, if possible, a mud or a peat bath. Nowadays, mud that has been imported in a concentrated form can be used in the bath at home, so that this therapy has been brought within the reach of everyone. It is also simple, and beneficial, to take an Epsom Salts bath or to relax the muscles and ligaments in a bath with bicarbonate of soda. Swimming in a heated pool is also an excellent form of exercise and I am delighted that, as a result of a renewed public interest, so many of the old and once-popular spas are again accessible to the public and all over the world thermal baths are being reopened or new ones are being established.

On a part-time basis I have a practice in a clinic in Arcen, in the southern part of the Netherlands. People travel there from far afield to bathe in the thermal waters which are pumped from a great depth. Their enthusiasm for this therapy is boundless, and many people have found relief from aches and pains, rheumatic complaints, nerve problems and blood circulatory and metabolic disorders.

The Institute of Medicine in Munich has recently completed an extensive study of balneotherapy and hydrotherapy, and their findings have justified many of the claims that are made in relation to these thermal baths throughout the world. They have confirmed that patients who suffer from the above-mentioned conditions are likely to benefit from the curative effects of the baths.

Many people have also found relief through herbal baths and in my book, *Water — Healer or Poison?*, detailed advice can be found on the many ways in which water can be used to improve one's health. Hot or cold sitz-baths or foot-baths will be helpful for a variety of health conditions, and if the water used contains minerals, so much the better.

Many patients have happily reported a considerable improvement since they decided to make a start with a multi-disciplinary programme, combining the use of the green-lipped mussel extract with hydrotherapy treatments. Even in the coldest winters, if the temperature of the water is maintained at a steady 34–5 °C (93–5 °F), people report a considerable reduction in pain. Sea-bathing is also an important form of hydrotherapy, but the climate in Northern Europe discourages most people from practising this on a round-the-year basis.

The French scientist, Louis Claude Vincent, was employed as an engineer by the French water authorities. During the twelve years he was in their employ he made an in-depth study of the water supply of thirty-two French towns. He found that in towns where the water originated from deep artesian wells in rocky regions and contained a high concentration of diluted minerals the overall mortality rate was low — between 615 and 900 per 100,000 inhabitants. However, where the people drank surface water that was chlorinated, the mortality rate rose sharply. These are interesting findings and they emphasise how important the quality of our water is. Water is not only a cleansing agent, it is also a great detoxifier and if water is pure it may be used effectively for this purpose. Blood tests taken from rheumatic and arthritic patients often show a high toxicity in the blood and I am convinced that water is a contributory factor to their condition. It is sad to say, but in my experience many arthritic and rheumatic patients live in areas where the public water supply is pumped through old lead pipes; as these pipes corrode, minimal lead poisoning results, which shows up in blood tests. Their crippling arthritic conditions might well have been avoided if their drinking water had come from a different supply system. Keeping our bodies clean is one thing, but ensuring that our water is clean is quite a feat nowadays, as pure and natural water is becoming an increasingly rare commodity.

—70 per cent of the weight of our brain is water;
—75 per cent of our muscles is water;
—83 per cent of our kidneys is water;
—22 per cent of our bones is water, and
—72 per cent of our blood consists of water.

Water plays an essential role in all the vital functions of the body: digestion, circulation, lubrication, elimination, absorption and regulation. Therefore we must endeavour to keep our water supply as pure and clean as possible.

Arthritic people are inclined towards poor blood circulation and many of my patients have been able to improve their conditions with water treatments.

One of the simplest methods is a form of hydrotherapy which at the clinic is often called "the cold dip". This is an exercise that should be done each morning on awakening and each evening when retiring. Place a basin of cold water at the side of the bed and keep a towel ready. On rising in the morning, place both feet in the water. After counting to ten, remove the feet from the water and place them on the towel. Exercise the toes as if trying to pick up a marble and do this ten to thirty times. Before going to bed at night, follow the same procedure. You will find that your feet are lovely and warm when you snuggle down in bed. The important thing to remember about this exercise is that it should be done for a minimum of sixty days to obtain the full benefit. As with some of the other water therapies mentioned, do not be fooled into thinking that this procedure is too simple to be effective, because I can assure you that, if you keep up the routine, you will experience considerable benefit.

Another excellent therapy is the hypothermic saltwater bath. This will help the heart, kidneys and also blood circulation and, again, it is of considerable benefit for rheumatic people. As the high density of salt in a hypothermic salt bath releases toxins from the skin, the patient should encourage this process through perspiration after taking the bath. For this purpose the patient will find it helpful to take a drink of hot herbal tea before going into the bath.

People who suffer from rheumatism should take a hypothermic saltwater bath once a week, if necessary. To prepare the bath, add 3 kg (6 lbs) of salt to a bath of comfortably warm water (36 °C/96.8 °F). Gradually increase the temperature of the water to approximately

105

44 °C (111 °F) over a period of twenty minutes. Immerse the body up to the neck and stay in the water for a period of 20–60 minutes, or as directed by your practitioner.

Do not rinse the body — only pat it dry, leaving the salt on the skin. Put on some warm nightclothes and immediately get into bed, covering yourself with a warm blanket and bedclothes. Stay in bed for one to two hours, or take the bath before retiring for the night. The body should subsequently be rinsed with fresh water to remove any toxins left on the skin.

Please note that it is recommended that someone be in attendance the first time a salt bath is taken and also that patients with heart or kidney problems should start with a lower water temperature. Sea salt or Epsom Salts may be used, or even bicarbonate of soda in some cases.

A hydrotherapy treatment or a visit to a thermal bath is of greater value than one could imagine and I am delighted that such methods are finding recognition once again. The Maoris must have known instinctively what health-giving properties their water possessed. According to their traditions, a waning moon was supposed to endow this living water with the gift of life to sustain them. With clever engineering work in the 1980s, some of those geysers in New Zealand have been adapted into hot pools or thermal baths and are available for public use. Natural springs, the world over, invariably contain some measure of medicinal value. The Maoris, however, rated theirs so highly because they claimed to receive extra strength from bathing in these waters.

Hydrotherapy, balneotherapy, Kneipp therapies and fangotherapies all have their value today. I cannot over-emphasise the tremendous healing power of water for rheumatic and arthritic people. Whether such therapies are taken at home, in the sea, in a thermal bath, or even in a sauna, the person concerned will always benefit.

# 8

## *Exercises*

WHEN GEORGE BERNARD SHAW visited Tikitere in New Zealand during his Dominion tour, he said that he was pleased to have the opportunity to get so close to Hades and yet be able to return — a privilege which he had never expected during his long life.

We can imagine why George Bernard Shaw reacted like this to the sights he must have seen. Not only can such thermal areas call up visions of hell with its "cauldrons", but it is more than likely that Shaw also witnessed some of the Maoris' tribal dances, and these too can be a fearsome sight. Thanks to the media, most of us will have had the opportunity to see a demonstration of some of these Maori dances, if only at the start of one of the rugby internationals or a state visit. Just imagine the impression left by such a performance in a landscape as witnessed by George Bernard Shaw!

What these dances clearly show, however, is that the Maoris must have been very fit and their stamina quite incredible. Their ability to dance so energetically is indicative of their fitness, but they were also known to cover large distances on foot and they fought many fierce battles, both on land and on water. They delighted in showing off their physical prowess and they would travel for days to tribal meetings where they could measure their strength against that of members from other tribes. Both men and women would attend such tribal gatherings. They could only have taken part in such demonstrations if they were in good physical health. We now know that the Maoris had all the prerequisites for good health at their fingertips, and from their history we learn that they took full advantage of them.

Exercises are very important to good health and there are a number of relaxation exercises that are of particular benefit to arthritic or rheumatic people. An excellent example of these is a breathing exercise practised according to the "Hara" technique. I have written about this exercise in my book *Stress and Nervous Disorders* and it is as easy as it is effective.

Lie flat on the floor and relax completely. Initially this may require a little practice, but persevere nevertheless. Close your eyes and tell every part of your body, from top to toe, to relax totally, until it feels as if your body is sinking deeper and deeper into the floor. Then place your left hand about half an inch beneath your navel and place your right hand over it. At that point, a magnetic ring on the vital centre of your being — "Hara" — will have been formed. It is at this centre that the vegetative nervous system is located. The Chinese believe that the navel is the gate to all happiness and certainly, by placing your hands in the position mentioned, you will feel completely relaxed. Next, breathe in slowly through the nose, filling your stomach with air and keeping your ribcage still. This sounds easier than it is, and it may well take a little time to master it properly.

Concentrate the mind on the stomach and breathe in slowly. Once the stomach is filled with air, round the lips and slowly breathe out, pulling the stomach flat. This can be done as often as you wish. Normally, the sensation after finishing this exercise is either one of complete relaxation and the desire for a nice sleep, or of refreshment and the desire to return to work. I must stress that it should be performed naturally, as a baby might do it. Sometimes it helps to imagine yourself walking in a beautiful garden where you discover the wonderful scent of roses, which you inhale slowly.

I have also described a number of exercises in my book *Neck and Back Problems*, but for arthritic people I would like here to highlight some that are particularly relevant, as this book is especially written with them in mind.

Lie flat on the floor on your back with your arms in a comfortable position alongside the body and do the following exercises:

—Bend your right knee and pull it up to your nose. Stretch the whole leg and lower it again. Repeat with the left leg.
—Do the same exercise with both legs at the same time.
—Bend your knees and place both feet flat on the floor. Now spread the knees and then close them again.
—Lift your right leg to as near a vertical position as possible and then lower it slowly. Repeat this with the left leg.
—Pull your knees up and place both feet flat on the floor. Stretch your arms sideways at an angle of ninety degrees. Keep both knees together and let them fall first to the left and then to the right. The hips are

109

allowed to rise off the floor, but the shoulders should remain flat on the floor.

Now turn over and lie face down, on your stomach, with your hands clasped in the small of your back, with your head resting on the floor.

—Raise your head and shoulders off the floor as far as possible. Lower and then rest them both before repeating several times.
—To continue on from the previous exercise, lift your head and shoulders and turn your head to the left and then to the right.
—Return to the starting position and stretch your arms alongside your body. Raise your left leg and then lower it again. Repeat with the right leg.
—For those people who are not too badly incapacitated, crawl along on your hands and knees. Try to do a little of this every day.
—Another useful exercise is to move your hips to the left and then to the right while standing up straight with your feet slightly apart. Take care to keep your shoulders still.
—Swing one arm round and round and follow this with the other arm.

Now for some exercises standing up straight, with your legs apart to the width of your shoulders.

—With your hands clasped loosely, bend forward and then backwards from the waist.
—Bending forward, dangle your head and arms loosely, as if they are hanging from a thread. Keeping your knees stretched, count to five and then return to starting position.

110

—Clench both hands tightly together and with your right leg stretched, lower your hands towards the left foot. Move the hands across the floor to the right foot, while stretching your left leg. Repeat this five times.

—Cross your arms in front of your chest, swing them together sideways, and then across in the opposite direction.

—Let your arms hang loosely beside your body, raise them up to shoulder level and down again. Try to bend your knees in rhythm with the arms.

—Hold on to the back of a chair or a high table. Swing your left leg forwards and backwards, and repeat with the other leg.

—Still standing in the same position, raise one leg out to the side, then lower it. Repeat with the other leg.

—This exercise can be done sitting down in order to loosen the arms. Pull your shoulders up towards your ears and then drop them down again, stretching the back and neck.

—Roll your shoulders round in circular movements, first forwards and then backwards.

—Bend your arms and raise your elbow sideways, then move them up and down several times.

—Place your hands at the back of the head or on the neck, bring your elbows forward and then stretch them backwards as far as possible.

Correct body posture is important, even when sitting down. To ensure that this is maintained at all times, try to adhere to the following advice.

—When driving a car, pull the seat forward and bend your knees. Ensure that the knees are higher than the hips. Sit up straight and place your hands high up on the steering wheel.

—When sitting in a wheelchair it is important that the seat of the chair is positioned as low as possible, and that both feet are supported by the foot rest. The knees should be higher than the hips, while making sure that the body is firmly supported by the back of the chair.

—Make sure that your bed has a good firm mattress.

—Walking is an excellent exercise, but make sure that your body is evenly balanced when walking.

—If there is an exaggerated hollow in the back, seek out a sturdy door. Stand up straight with your back against the door, ensuring that your heels, calves, back, shoulders and head are all in touch with the door. Then slide down, keeping your back against the door, and then slide up again back to the starting position. Repeat this up and down movement several times.

—When sitting at rest, it is beneficial to position one foot higher than the other.

—When bending, always bend at the knees. The chest should come down, and the underarms will often touch the knees.

—When lifting, make sure that your back remains straight and always lift by bending at the knees, keeping the knees together. Never lift more weight than you can comfortably manage.

—It is best to carry the same weight in each hand when shopping or travelling. I travel frequently and I often see elderly people struggling at airports or railway stations. When carrying heavy luggage, people rarely notice whether they are evenly laden, i.e. if the case in one hand is of comparable weight to the luggage in the other hand.

—Arthritic people should realise how important it is that their joints are regularly exercised, even though this may be a painful process. Lack of movement causes the condition to deteriorate more rapidly.

—Massage, reflexology or aromatherapy can bring relief, as those methods affect every part of the body: the glands, organs, tissue, circulation, limbs, muscles and nerves.

—Steam baths, saunas and whirlpools are effective and these practices can form part of an overall fitness programme for mind, body and spirit.

Unfortunately, there are many reasons why our energy flow can become obstructed. Often, there is no obvious reason. However, there are many ways to avoid such a situation. First of all, try and remain as active as possible. Take physical exercise in the fresh air: go swimming, walking or take up cycling. Do not overdo it, but plan your exercise. In particular, never overdo a certain exercise if it makes you uncomfortable.

Relaxation is also a very important part of the treatment for rheumatic and arthritic people. Again, there are certain exercises which encourage relaxation, such as autogenic training, the "Hara" breathing method or visualisation techniques. The most important thing is to allow yourself plenty of rest.

Try to go out into the fresh air and, if possible, enjoy the sunshine. Dry temperatures are often invigorating and although a change of temperature will not do any harm, many arthritic people feel much better in dry heat. Hot and cold temperature variations are not necessarily detrimental for arthritic conditions, and it is not recommended that the arthritic patient stay in the heat all the time. Most arthritic people thrive on sunshine, for its pleasant warmth and the dry air, while the ultra-violet light from the sun is good for our skin. It also encourages calcium metabolism, which is always under threat in arthritic people or those affected by osteoporosis. But be sensible about sunbathing. Frequent sunbathing is important, but do not overdo it. The best times are between nine and eleven in the morning and after two o'clock in the afternoon, and fifteen minutes to half an hour is really sufficient. It will benefit the skin, the muscles and ligaments.

So, we have now established that a balanced programme of rest, exercise and relaxation is important. If possible, enquire about physiotherapy, hydrotherapy and the extremely relaxing thermal bathing. Above all, avoid the stress of working more than eight hours a day and take a rest at regular intervals. Work towards a happy and low-stress working environment. Keep moving, while also allowing time for sufficient and worthwhile relaxation. Cultivate a creative hobby, such as playing a musical instrument, painting or even gardening. Think about your diet and make any necessary changes in accordance with my earlier advice. Do not forget that emotional worries are likely to exacerbate your physical problems.

Consider the lifestyle of the Maoris: they entertained themselves with dancing, singing and swimming, and they lived in harmony with nature. Here is a lesson for us to learn. We too could move a bit closer to nature and take some responsibility for our health, and I am sure that after only a brief period, we would begin to appreciate the results.

# 9

## Research

DO WE REALLY understand the whole picture of arthritis and rheumatism? I would immediately respond to such a question by posing another one of my own: do the medical specialists fully understand the immune system or the endocrine system?

There are too many unexplained mysteries in the human body for us to believe that the medical profession has more than a few partially effective ideas about treating the immune system. We know that if we are lucky enough to be able to pinpoint the specific cause of a lack of immunity, it is generally possible to effect a recovery. Yet too many mysteries still remain. This is also true of the endocrine system. The endocrinologist can explain the presence of certain conditions as being the result of hormonal imbalances, yet although we have learned much, no one would dare to claim full understanding of this intricate system. Recently, it has been recognised that rheumatism and arthritis are somehow connected to both the immune and endocrine systems.

In alternative medicine, we endeavour to approach such problems from the holistic point of view: to study mind, body and spirit as three integral and interrelated parts of one and the same entity. At present, I am spending a fair amount of time on certain research projects, and my starting point is always to consider mental and emotional influences, as well as the symptomatic condition. No doubt it is easier to take note of the symptoms and use this information as the basis for deciding on a course of treatment. It is much more time-consuming, yet infinitely more interesting, to relate any local complaint of illness to the wider spectrum of the whole person and, bearing all this in mind, devise an appropriate treatment programme.

I would respectfully refuse to estimate the number of people currently receiving treatment for rheumatism and arthritis, the cause of whose affliction can be traced back to an emotional trauma, nor, for that matter, how many people are under treatment because of a hormonal imbalance caused by an internal disharmony of some kind.

What do we think of a possible connection between colours and the endocrine glands? In certain circles it is believed that the pineal gland reacts to violet colours, the eyes to greenish-blue, the thymus gland to yellow, the gonads to red, and so on. Let me remind you of the significance of the number seven: there are seven endocrine glands, seven colours in the solar spectrum, and also seven layers of light receptors in the retina of the eye. Harmony in colour, or for that matter the lack of it, relates to a corresponding balance in our physical condition.

Illness and disease are disharmony and in this context every aspect of health must be considered. A minor factor could cause disharmony and therefore in our research we must consider all possibilities in our search for a chemical balance or imbalance. In earlier chapters I have frequently mentioned that worthwhile marine product, the extract of the green-lipped mussel. In nature everything is a matter of balance. Seawater, as part of our natural environment, is subject to this law also. Seawater can sometimes have great healing powers. Please do not correct me by saying that I should speak in the past tense, because I will not accept that we will not soon wake up to our responsibilities and learn to protect our environment from polluting influences.

It is sometimes considered ill-judged to refer to the body as a chemical laboratory, yet if the body is healthy, it is chemically balanced. If the body is mentally, emotionally and physically in balance, then there is health. Much depends on what I call the "pillars of health": nutrition, digestion, elimination, circulation and relaxation.

Nutrition depends on good digestion through the mouth, the stomach and the duodenum. In turn, this is dependent on the presence of amino acids, glucose, essential fatty acids, enzymes, vitamins, minerals and oxygen, which are all needed to allow maximum absorption. Good absorption will break down and apportion nutrients to the blood, liver, heart and organ cells. Balance in this context means that waste material is able to leave the body and the waste material in the blood can be eliminated through the kidneys, lungs and skin. Effective elimination has been recognised as a significant factor because arthritic and rheumatic people are often plagued by constipation. Residual waste must be encouraged to leave the body at regular intervals.

The Maoris set great store by relaxation. It is evident from their rituals, their games and other activities, that they understood the art of relaxation. Unfortunately, for many of us today this is no longer the case, as at any stage of our lives we can be pushed or driven hard to become high achievers, usually at the expense of relaxation. Even in our sports this competitive element has become predominant. Don't let anyone fool you into believing that professional sports people are relaxed in their efforts to excel. Whilst sport is supposed to be a means of relaxation, for many of us the determination to win and the drive required to do so renders it a worthless pastime as an exercise in relaxation.

In the analytical diagnostic approach to rheumatism and arthritis, responding with some standard form of treatment should be avoided. A correct analysis can only be reached after having taken account of blood tests, allergy checks and the condition of the auto-immune system. Most patients clearly benefit from a cleansing course, after which a programme can be started which includes some herbal remedies. The criteria to be established beforehand are the degree or presence of stiffness, pain, swelling, nodules, deformation of the joints, fluid retention, histological changes and long-term complaints. A range of therapies may be advised, such as manipulation, acupuncture, mineral baths and exercises. From my research I have concluded that it is important to widen the programme options as much as possible.

I recently heard a rheumatologist state categorically that diet has no bearing whatsoever on rheumatic and arthritic conditions. Sadly, this is not the case. From my own research I have concluded that the direct opposite is true, and in particular the balance between carbohydrates and proteins — acid and alkaline — is of great importance. We are also told that worry and stress are natural and that trauma is part of our natural make-up, and these factors are claimed to have no bearing on rheumatism and arthritis. Yet, we know that these factors not only deplete the immune system, but also result in a lack of strength. I have even seen the effects of excessive jealousy and possessiveness influence a person's condition adversely. It shows a lack of understanding to say that such emotions cannot physically influence a person. Even the smallest negative vibration influences the vital force in a person. Patients are often told after an illness that as soon as he or she has gained some strength, everything will be all right. How can we regain our strength if the blood circulation is inadequate? This causes a lack of strength in every part of our body. After each attack of so-called sickness, no matter how minor, the body's vitality, supplied by the blood, will have been weakened, and this weakness, in turn, will cause congestion in our back, hips and lower limbs.

I have sometimes been criticised for my statements on negative vibration. However, the conscious system accepts vibrations, either negative or positive, just as the physical body absorbs water. Likewise, food enters our stomach, yet people often allow their conscious system to become contaminated by worries about the calories contained in food. Fears and worries are likely to act as negative vibrations. It is true, for example, that small indications such as flatulence caused by worry, or diarrhoea caused by fear of examinations, will travel upwards from the stomach to the brain — and we must understand that the human body absorbs vibrations just as a sponge absorbs water.

The human body is a perfect, but very peculiar, structure. It seems strange that there are as many bones and joints in our feet as there are in the whole of our spine, from the atlas to the end of the coccyx. Yet, the spinal

119

cord, with its various branches, must help to supply all the different parts of the body. Remember too that life depends on the blood and the blood depends on the glandular system for its support. As each set of glands contributes different secretions to the blood, so our glands should be given just as much, if not more, consideration than the blood itself. This is the reason why we must provide the endocrine glands not only with the nutrients they need, but also with mental stimulation. I have sometimes referred to the endocrine glands as "the glands that treat mind, body and soul", and this explains why imagination and visualisation therapy can be of such great benefit in the treatment of many patients.

The imagination is based in the subconscious part of the brain. When a view or image is visualised in goodness and subsequently projected to all parts of the body, there is harmony. If one imagines evil or sadness, these will soon be manifested. In the same way, by applying the law of universal knowledge, detrimental objects and causes can be removed from the body's organs. If a man imagines that he is suffering from some undesirable condition in his body or brain and allows these thoughts to enter his subconscious, he may well begin to experience the relevant symptoms. Or vice versa, he can use the same power to influence a good or a sound part of the brain or body. This phenomenon can apply to toothache as well as cancer. By the same power such troubles can be removed if the law is correctly applied.

Thought is often stronger than matter, and we have to learn to visualise this perfect harmony within ourselves. In the same way we can learn to recognise the difference between material knowledge and spiritual knowledge. It is good to identify that part of man that exists in the material world and also the part that belongs to the spiritual world. The material side of man is the centre of the conscious system and in many cases our sickness, worry, fear and discontent are caused by interference in this part of our being.

Often, these emotions cause an imbalance in the endocrine system. For instance, it is staggering to see how many imbalances can be caused by thyroid problems. If the hormones produced by the thyroid glands are hindered in their movement, they can turn into poison. The thyroid gland is of great importance to us, more so than most people realise.

In the chapter on vitamins, minerals and trace elements, we have seen that when the hormones have been separated, they pass from each side of our throat to the heart. It appears that in these lobes, hormones of a different kind are produced. The main hormone resembles iodine, while another hormone contains a small percentage of sulphuric acid. Nature has equipped the thyroid gland with a hormone that is necessary for purifying the blood to a certain consistency before it enters our heart. When the actions and functions of the glands of our body are properly understood and these glands are adequately nourished, mentally and physically, they can be restored to perfect function and in a perfect world they will provide every substance that is required for a healthy body.

Now let us look at the kidneys, or the adrenal glands, which also form part of the endocrine system. The urinary system is frequently a source of problems for arthritic and rheumatic people. This system eliminates not only the waste fluids from our body, but also eliminates much of the body's broken down minerals and tissues. When people speak of the urinary organs they think of the kidneys, the urethra and the bladder. These organs form a complicated network that draws the waste matter from every part of our body, with the exception of the fluid which is eliminated through the sweat glands or pores in the skin. Of course, the bladder is the main reservoir for this fluid after the body has taken what it needs. Cell tissue in the kidneys also does important work, and there is also a gland attached to each kidney, located immediately above and in front of the upper end of the kidney, called the adrenal or suprarenal glands. These adrenal glands produce two or three hormones, some of which neutralise substances as they enter the kidney and separate and break down waste matter from the blood. The kidney filters all this refuse into large tubes known as the ureters, which extend down into the bladder at the lower extremity of the body. The adrenal hormones stimulate the tissue and the action of our kidneys when the glands are in perfect working order. They also stimulate the action of the blood as it leaves the kidneys and the blood conveys this stimulation to the heart. Harmony in the endocrine system is of the greatest importance and even these small adrenal glands should work in harmony with the rest of the endocrine glands.

So far, little research has been undertaken on the pituitary and the pineal glands. In general, little attention is paid to the pituitary gland, yet a finely tuned balance between this gland and the pineal gland is tremendously important. Mental and physical harmony must be restored when disease or illness rules the body.

I have said before that the hormones produced by these glands pass directly into our bloodstream in order to renew the life and vigour of our body. In the absence of any one of these hormones the blood also becomes imbalanced.

The pituitary produces various kinds of hormone. One of these contributes to the regulation of blood pressure; another rebuilds the blood vessels and renews veins that have been destroyed by tubercular conditions; a further hormone increases the supply of fluid to the spinal column and simultaneously increases the action of the urine and the hormones of the adrenals when they are active. Yet another pituitary hormone has a stimulating effect on the tissues of the smooth muscles of our body, especially the uterine muscles causing contraction, and is essential for the bladder and the reproductive organs to work properly. The pituitary also secretes a substance which has a strong influence on the thyroid, the adrenal glands and the regulation of the growth of the skeleton.

When the pituitary gland is inactive, the face, hands or feet often swell. Sometimes this can signal the beginning of a rheumatic condition. Often when the gland is inactive it will swell, thereby placing pressure on the optic nerve and causing a specific type of blindness. As the face becomes bloated, many different disturbances in the head can occur, which may cause headaches. So, we can begin to understand that this apparently insignificant gland has an enormous responsibility; just as the exact octave is required in a harmonious melody, this gland should be in optimum working order to best serve the body.

Less research still has been undertaken into the pineal gland, which produces a number of different mineral substances that cannot be replaced by material substances. The analysis which is given in the twenty-third edition of *Gray's Anatomy* (page 1,266) is as follows: "In our research work we find that the pineal gland produces and stimulates seven different minerals in the human body. Much of this action is carried out by the spinal column."

We know that the body is dependent on various phosphates, magnesium, calcium, etc., hence the importance of minerals. In experiments on the spinal column the spinal cord has been punctured and fluid has been extracted to determine the course of different ailments. On many occasions these experiments have resulted in the loss of the use of lower limbs. Also, air has been injected into the spinal cord. The air naturally works its way up the spinal cord to the brain, exerting pressure on the voluntary nervous system and causing the flesh to become hard.

As an osteopath I know only too well how much trouble can be caused by the displacement of bones in the neck, when the neck becomes twisted and out of alignment, impinging on the spinal cord, so that the circulation to the body below the shoulders is obstructed. This causes a deficiency of nerve energy in the spinal cord which, in turn, causes it to become limp. This then allows the bones of the spine to move out of position, which is the beginning of problems too numerous to mention. When the spinal column is impaired, the resulting restriction of the blood circulation often leads to some form of paralysis or arthritis. Meanwhile, as the pineal gland continues to produce hormones, and the circulation in the spinal cord is obstructed, the pineal gland becomes swollen or enlarged and this interferes with the function of the ventricles of the brain, the body's regulatory action, the medulla and many other bodily functions. It also places an unnatural pressure on the nerves to the eyes and ears.

The pineal gland is susceptible to cosmic energy. If we lay ourselves open to the negative influences of cosmic energy or we are chained to a word processor or television screen, we lower the efficiency of the immune system, as the pineal gland becomes affected and will in turn affect the immune system through its ally, the thymus gland.

One school of thought favours the removal of the thymus gland, especially for the treatment of the condition affecting the muscles known as myasthenia gravis. At birth the thymus gland may be only the size of a pea, while by the age of about forty, it will already have decreased in size. Yet that minute thymus gland will continue to perform its function until the day we die, and sometimes it is even given the label of the "gland of immunity". This indeed is praise! The thymus gland can even affect the voice. We sometimes hear of famous singers suffering from recurrent throat problems and losing control of their voice. Only recently I treated a well-known broadcaster for throat problems by stimulating the thymus function. The thymus gland has a direct connection with the red blood corpuscles, the heart and the spleen, and inhibition of the red corpuscles proves the distinct connection with the veins and arteries of the body. It is my belief that if we knew more about the working of the thymus gland, a state of perfect health could be achieved. Unfortunately, the importance of this gland is very much underrated and this does nothing to alleviate the suffering of arthritic or rheumatic people. Remember that it was this gland that was considered worthy of the name "gland of immunity".

The pancreas is yet another endocrine gland and a healthy balanced diet will encourage this gland to produce the important pancreatic enzymes which are so essential for overall health. These digestive enzymes are crucial because the incorrect breakdown of ingested fats, proteins and sugars can lead to digestive complaints. The islets of Langerhans — a group of cells within the pancreas — secrete insulin into the blood and so influence the level of glucose in the body. The pancreas also plays an important role in regulating the body's normal balance.

At present I am involved in a research project, the aim of which is to identify the essential balance of the various glands of the endocrine system for arthritic and rheumatic people. I sometimes think of the traditional ways of the Maoris, and how their physical and mental characteristics and lifestyle involuntarily stimulated these glands. It appears to me that they had found a good harmony between mind and body and this was expressed in their respect for each other. It can often be observed in supposedly less-civilised societies than ours, that the endocrine system reacts positively to mutual love, respect and harmony. Whereas we in the West live in a materialistic world beset with stress, worries and fears, people such as the Maoris who lived closer to nature, show us that universal love is in no way connected with an individual's passion. Universal love is that emotion exemplified in "Love thy neighbour as thyself" and this portrays itself in improved physical harmony.

Circulation is another "pillar of health", and is especially relevant in arthritic conditions. In one of my earlier books, *Heart and Blood Circulatory Problems*, I have concentrated on this aspect of physical health. How can we promote more effective circulation?

Our food intake stimulates the blood to a certain extent and when the nutrients obtained from our food are combined with the red and white cells and tissues, the body tissue becomes stronger and increases our vitality. When the veins and arteries are free from problems, allowing the blood to circulate without interference as it passes through the lungs, retaining the little molecules of iron, this produces heat and vitality in every part of the body.

Normal blood circulation takes about three minutes from the time the blood leaves the heart to when it returns to the lungs, having made a complete revolution of the body. Free-flowing circulation is of great importance; the large veins on the outer part of our body are not as easily congested as those deep inside the body. The more congestion in the flesh, the harder and more congested the body becomes, and the more pressure is raised in the inner circulation. This causes the body to age prematurely and become sluggish. Lack of heat in the blood also prevents the hormones from working effectively.

The blood circulatory system resembles a hot-water or central-heating system. It is supposed to furnish heat to all parts of our body, thereby enabling the digestive juices to flow freely and facilitating the action of the digestive tracts, as well as that of the elimination process. We should never allow our blood count to become low or irregular. If both the blood and the red corpuscles appear to be weak, they can be strengthened. Similarly, if the pulse is fast and jerky, it means that the spine, shoulders, neck and arms need treatment.

The heart is merely a pump composed of muscles, fibrous tissue and elastic fibre. If the neck, shoulders and arms are kept in good condition, there will be no trouble with the heart. If the spine, hips and lower limbs are working properly and freely without any tension, aches and pains, the blood will be able to circulate more freely and so will relieve any pressure. If the circulation is normal the heart will carry out its duties quietly and smoothly, so that we will seldom give any thought to this organ. The condition of the blood influences our disposition, which changes as our blood changes.

We should realise that blood is the motor power of the body and that it is impossible to move a leg or raise an arm until the force of blood penetrates that part of the body. Take, for instance, the paralytic or arthritic patient, whose blood circulation in the limbs experiences some obstruction. Why is it so difficult for an arthritic person to move the limbs affected in this way? Because there is insufficient blood in those parts to furnish the motor power that is necessary. That brings us back to the glandular system, which influences such a vast area of our health.

Now for another brief look at two other glands that form part of the endocrine system, i.e. the pineal gland and the pituitary gland. There is little doubt that the pineal gland or "third eye", as it is sometimes called, is definitely influenced by stress, prayer and meditation. At the same time it is true that we don't yet know enough about the medical or physical aspect of the pineal gland. This gland, by means of acupuncture, can be balanced positively or negatively. When treating stress-related conditions, working on this particular gland can sometimes produce very rewarding results.

The pituitary gland is said to be the key to the chemistry of the whole of the body. The pituitary hormones chemically affect the cell membranes, therefore the chemical reactions do not work properly when the pituitary gland is in any way impaired. A good intake of protein or, more specifically, good vegetable protein, is most important for the production of hormones and also the different enzymes in the body. If the body's enzyme production is insufficient, the hormone balance will fail to meet the requirements of a healthy immune system.

The pituitary gland is also often referred to as the "master gland" or "conductor of the orchestra", and it releases hormones whose function is either to promote or inhibit the release of other endocrine hormones. Indirectly, it controls such basic processes as rate of growth, metabolic rate, water and electrolyte balance, kidney filtration, ovulation and lactation. It responds to hormones released by the region of the brain known as the hypothalamus, and is a physical link between the nervous and the endocrine system.

The divisions of the heart, the arteries and the ventricles, are all subject to order and disorder. The liver is like a complicated laboratory with connections leading to the gall bladder, from there to the stomach, and from the stomach down to the duodenum. The condition and functional efficiency of these organs and glands are significant indications in the drive towards rebuilding and establishing a permanently healthy body.

I often carry out a thorough examination of the throat and tonsils when checking over arthritic or rheumatic patients. In this situation I am extremely grateful to the elderly doctor who showed me, many years ago, how to perform acupuncture in the throat. So often a crippling arthritic problem has been triggered by a tonsil condition, or in some cases because of some malfunction of the salivary glands, which play a major role in the digestion of food. A dry mouth or tongue, or a rasping sensation when swallowing food may be overcome by regulating the salivary glands. A distended or congested neck can be responsible for these conditions, as the main body of the salivary glands is located in the cheek, just in front of the ear. A tube-like gland extends from the upper part of the main salivary gland on the side of the face which connects with the mouth, close to the tonsil. The lower salivary glands extend forward into the cavity of the lower jaw, connecting with the roots of the tongue. The flow of saliva can be regulated by working on the roots of the tongue. During treatment, the tongue should be pressed firmly against the bottom of the mouth, so that the tongue lies flat. Turn the tip of the tongue back until it comes into contact with the cord that holds the tongue in place. Then press very gently and saliva will begin to flow immediately.

The next consideration must be our tonsils. These are constructed of lymphoid tissue and produce an oily substance, and their importance should not be under-estimated. One of their duties is to protect the stomach, with which they have a direct connection. If we eat some food that may make us feel nauseous, or that may cause poisoning, the tonsils warn us by sending hormones through a small tube to the stomach. In many cases this will result in the stomach dispelling the detrimental food through vomiting. The salivary glands and the tonsils also constitute an important part of the lymphatic system, which is responsible for fending off many illnesses. We must always bear in mind that the actions of the hormones produced by the salivary glands and the tonsils are essential to our health and this brings us straight to the importance of the lymphatic system.

The number of lymphatic vessels in the body is far higher than the arteries and veins taken together, and these lymphatic vessels have connections with all parts of the internal organs. They lie underneath the skin and the scalp and have a strong influence on the thyroid gland. They carry the sense actions to all parts of the body; for example, the sense of taste, good or bad, is affected by the condition of the lymph. The lymph influences the action of any part of the neck and hands, and if the lymph becomes thick and sluggish, it gradually slows down the flow of the blood, as the gland supplies strength to the red blood cells. The more active the lymph becomes, the more quickly the body will move.

The lymphatic system consists of a complex network of connected vessels which collect the lymph from various organs and tissues of the human body and conduct it to the large veins of the neck, connecting with the jugular vein and other less important veins, where the lymph is discharged into the bloodstream. Within this system of connecting vessels there are many lymph glands or nodes. These little nodes or sacs, which act as filters and separate one substance from another, resemble buttons on a string, and are positioned at varying distances apart.

We will start with head and face and draw an imaginary line from the back of the throat to the third cervical vertebra located in the middle of the neck. Here we find these strings of lymphatic nodes extending from the deeper tissue and travelling through the flesh on the face and head beneath the skin. One branch occupying the skin travels up the jaw to the eye, while two other branches travel to the nose. Two important nodes lie between the ear and the cheekbone, along a line from the ear to the tip of the nose. From here the glands, fifteen or twenty in number, travel to both sides of the head. The function of these glands is to collect fats and waste material and carry them into deeper portions of the body. Just above the collarbone on either side of the neck we find another group of these little nodes, five or six on either side, extending down into the deeper part of the body and yet more branches extend to the flesh and connect with the shoulders. You can feel these little nodes in many parts of the body.

The next major group is located in the back of the neck, travelling up inside the skull, where it acts as a drainage system, and continues from there down to the lower part of the body. The heat ratio of our body depends greatly on the action of these lymphatic nodes. Elderly people who are troubled with a cold sensation on the back of the neck, just at the base of the skull, should place their right hand on the back of the neck covering the area that feels cold. Within a short time they will feel a new vigour and circulation in the flesh and skin, which in time will eradicate any deeply grooved wrinkles on the back of the neck.

We will now direct our attention to the lymphatic system of the neck, starting beneath the skin, which travels

along the two main arteries down to the breastbone —
the sternum. This group of lymphatics again can be
likened to buttons on a string, descending from the
collarbone to the solar plexus. There is also a little string
of lymph nodes that extends from the spinal column,
sending out connecting branches to the various parts of
the flesh and diaphragm. Going back to just below the
collarbone, we will find a large knot with branches run-
ning in different directions beneath the flesh extending
into the armpits. From there many lymphatic veins travel
down both arms, but the largest groups are to be found in
the palms of the hands and the fingers. Here we notice
the relation between the lymphatic group and the conscious system which carries the sense of vibration. All
that is necessary to trace the lymphatics is to draw one
finger of the right hand along the corresponding finger
on the opposite hand and you experience the sensation
of "touch".

This feeling is very important, because the next group of
lymphatics, extending from the shoulders down towards
the trunk of the body, with branches going to the breast,
is sited deeper in the flesh. The entire breast is one solid
network of glands, with the exception of the nipples. This
network of lymphatics influences the mammary glands.
In the lower part of the lumbar region we find a large
lymphatic gland that is similar to an artery. At this point
the gland branches out into a dozen or so nodes. In the
female, other little strings of nodes extend into the lower
part of the body, to the fallopian tubes, the ovarian glands,
the uterus, the vagina and lower limbs. These glands
collect the lymph from the lower extremities and carry
it in the direction of the heart. There it connects with
one of the main arteries and pours the lymph and chyle
— a milk-like substance — into the blood. The lymph
is circulated with the blood until it passes through the

kidneys, where any detrimental substances are extracted and then eliminated by the urinary channels.

Usually, any problem with the lymphatic system can be treated using simple remedies like Dr Vogel's Kelpasan (extract of sea kelp) and Urticalcin (a calcium preparation); these can be used to reduce any swelling of the lymph glands through the assistance they give to the body's elimination process. Often when I see that waste material remains within the lymphatic system and is not eliminated, I deduce that the adenoids or the sinuses have become involved.

One always has to be careful with swollen lymph glands because even a draught of cold air striking the nostrils can cause a chill to run over the entire body. This sends a shiver through the body and sometimes the adenoids are affected. Yet it is important that the adenoids function properly. The same goes for the sinuses, which also play an important role in protecting the body against rheumatism and arthritis. We must never forget that each system of the body has its own function and tasks to perform, and this fact should be borne in mind should we be tempted to have the adenoids or tonsils removed, or to indulge in sinus washes.

The sinus system of the human head acts as a ventilation system. One of its duties is to restore oxygen to the different tissues of the brain, and then to collect refuse from the head and expel it from the frontal sinuses into the nostrils. The sphenoedal sinus is located behind the nostrils, close to the pituitary gland and at times it appears to drain the surplus and detrimental mucus from the inner part of the head. An opening in the frontal bone of the sphenoedal sinus allows this discharge to enter the cavity of the nostril. In many cases of sinus disorders the mucus travels down from the nostrils to the throat,

133

causing the person affected to produce a phlegm-like mucus. So, you will now realise why it is important that the sinuses are kept clear.

A little stiffness in the neck, or soreness if the middle bone of the neck is displaced out of alignment, can interfere with the teeth by restricting the circulation and nerve energy, causing the teeth to decay and develop infections which may eventually result in rheumatism or arthritis.

Seemingly trivial or minor problems should always be investigated. This advice may sound over-cautious but nevertheless it should be heeded. This is the time to stop minor problems from developing into major ones. We should learn a few simple lessons from nature and for that, fortunately, a brilliant brain is not necessary.

We will learn as we go along how to deal with certain things that have to be done in any event. Potential infections stemming from viruses or bacteria can result in major problems and the use of neural therapy to overcome these has been well researched. This method is used to find the source of the infection and if the infection is still active it can be treated by injection. Research into neural therapy is still ongoing and, fortunately, in many hospitals and clinics this method is achieving greater recognition.

Good results have also been obtained with enzyme therapy, which is also given by injection in the form of Rheumajecta, an injection of anti-inflammatory enzymes. At a recent seminar, where both orthodox and natural treatments were discussed following a series of trials, and where the rheumatologists present were able to compare notes, it was concluded that with a multi-disciplinary programme with which the trials were conducted, tremendous benefits can be obtained from this therapy.

I would insist that the living conditions in those countries where, even today, arthritis is unknown should be the subject of greater study. Remember the ways of the Maoris and just think how much cheaper and cost-effective it would be if we could reduce our dependence on tremendously expensive drugs. Health problems could be drastically reduced by the introduction of a healthy diet, supplementary vitamins, minerals and trace elements, and products such as green-lipped mussel, Imperarthritica and some of the herbal preparations from Heath and Heather. Indeed, I was staggered by some of the statistics I learned from my own country. The Netherlands has approximately fifteen million inhabitants, and a breakdown of expenditure on national health care shows that approximately £1.6 million per hour is spent on hospital beds, blood transfusions, drugs, bandages and plasters. This money has to be earned by the people themselves. Would it not make more sense to re-educate people towards exerting greater self-discipline and learning to care for themselves while showing more respect for their health?

The World Health Organisation has declared a laudable aim: health for all by the year 2000. I am sure that this goal can only be realised if each individual is prepared to shoulder the responsibility for his or her own actions. The Maoris probably did this in a very simple way, but one which is no longer practicable under the present environmental circumstances. We know that the occurrence of chronic illnesses, and especially rheumatism and arthritis, is ever-increasing. The quality of life for rheumatic people is clearly much reduced: tiredness, stiffness and dysfunction takes its toll. Remember that although some of the methods discussed in this book are simple, this does not mean that they are not effective.

## BY APPOINTMENT ONLY

As far as the aim of the World Health Organisation is concerned international co-operation will be necessary, and in order to alleviate human suffering we cannot afford to overlook or write off any method which can successfully reduce the pain, or limit the occurrence of, these crippling disabilities.

# 10

## *Conclusion*

THIS BOOK PRESENTS a crystallised view of the Maori lifestyle. Together we have looked into the past, a few centuries ago. Personally, I have thoroughly enjoyed reading up on the habits, rituals and the health of the Maori people. Once again it has left me with a few thought-provoking ideas and I would like to think that we have all learned something that may well lead us to a better quality of health, especially for those readers who suffer from arthritic or rheumatic disorders.

The Maoris have always fascinated me. For reasons I have already explained, the island of Mokoia fascinates me even more. It was, after all, a New Zealand patient who told me that the original island of Mokoia is also referred to as "the Island of Love". I hope that those people who have experienced a period of rest and respite in our Scottish Mokoia, on the boundaries of one of the world's famous golf courses, overlooking the majestic views of the setting sun over the hills of the beautiful island of Arran, will remember that time with fondness.

The island of Mokoia in New Zealand is steeped in history. It is an island of great beauty and at one time a good quality of life was enjoyed there — a healthy life, a life free of arthritic pain. Perhaps our western culture owes the Maoris a greater debt than we had previously realised for having inflicted "civilisation" upon them. For there is no doubt that the adoption of our ways has been detrimental to their healthy existence.

In the Scottish clinic of Mokoia many rheumatic and arthritic patients have found a way to control their debilitating condition and a good many of them have even found a cure. Many of them have written to me with glowing testimonies about the success of their programmes. I will always remember, gratefully and fondly, the elderly lady who first told me about the green-lipped mussel extract. Nowadays, a large number of my patients are able to benefit from this wonderful remedy without which I would not have been able to help so many arthritic people. This lady found the ultimate cure for her arthritic condition, and she still speaks with amazement of the period of her recovery.

I have managed to trace back the history of the Mokoia residence only as far as the last century or so, and even at that time it was known by its present name. Because of its renewed link with its roots, I will always think of it as the best place I have ever visited.

I often think with envy of the Maori culture, envy for their healthy constitution until they became attracted to some of our Western ways and habits. It was not until the late 1860s that the first signs of colonisation began to take effect. It was at that time too when Father Mahoney of Taronga claimed to have found a cure for rheumatism in a thermal pool — and a spa was born. Today, we know that there is much more to be learned from the Maori lifestyle and I have set out to tell you about some of their ways in this book.

If we look at what we introduced these people to, we must conclude that coffee, for example, has not stood them in good stead — and the same applies to many of our other customs. Our diet, with its high proportion of starches and animal proteins, has created problems for the Maoris as well as for us. Alcohol has proved to be harmful to these people — as it has in our culture. Excess toxicity resulting from eating the wrong foods has led to a deterioration in the Maoris' health and they have become vulnerable to diseases which have long been rife in our civilisation, but which were unheard of in their own. Genetics play a major role in illness patterns and I wonder what the future will bring.

Remember how careful the Maoris were in the preparation of their food and how they refused even to touch food with unclean hands. Instinctively, they knew not to combine certain foods. We must believe that returning to a correct diet will restore some of that lost health. The popularity of fast food has caused many problems in New Zealand, as it has elsewhere. At lectures or public meetings I am often asked if we have reached the point of no return. I believe that we have been given a great challenge to show that it can be done differently, even in today's society. Many of the patients who have attended the Mokoia clinic in Scotland and whom I have encouraged to consider certain dietary changes, are to this day still grateful for the help and the relief they have experienced, and treasure their new-found freedom and mobility.

From Maori legends it becomes clear that the island of Mokoia was considered as the pearl in the crown for the early Maoris and considerable subterfuge has taken place

139

since its discovery. This feat has been claimed by various chiefs and disputes concerning the right to live on the island has caused considerable rivalry. Earlier I mentioned the Maoris' devotion to Te Matua-tonga, a kumara god and a stone emblem of fertility. A well-known saying, indicating the power they accorded to Te Matua-tonga, was *"Kia tu tangatanga te aro ki Mokoia"* — "Let the way be open to Mokoia".

A historian with a special affinity for the Maoris, James Cowan, recorded the following song:

> *Who will feast upon*
> *The stores of dried fish yonder?*
> *The throats of the people of Mokoia,*
> *The place of the well-filled ovens,*
> *Will be a relish for us*
> *To go down with the kumara.*
> *Aha! How sweet it will be.*

Despite their apparent abundance of food, they never seemed to have taken this for granted. The above song shows their appreciation of the two main sources of food — fish in any shape or form and the kumara, their much-loved sweet potato. In combination with their other dietary habits and methods of food preparation, these foods gave the Maoris a well-balanced diet, which is so important to prevent degenerative diseases.

There is a balance to be found in nature, as there is in the sea, and although that balance may shift at times, let us please try not to lose it. Remember the three forms of energy: food, water and air. If we want better general health and are prepared to shoulder the responsibility of working towards it, we must also realise that we have to protect these forms of sources of life, keeping them as pure and unspoilt as possible.

If for any reason your health is affected, please do not give in by telling yourself, or for that matter letting anyone else tell you, that you will have to learn to live with it. Don't follow that road, because it just is not true! You owe it to yourself and you owe it to those who love you to do all that is possible to bring about a change. We must sever the link between pollution and allergies, bearing in mind that allergic reactions contribute towards degeneration. Today, rheumatism and arthritis occur the world over. What are we going to do about it?

To me it is quite clear. I have visited so-called Third World countries, where people can still remember when arthritis and rheumatism were unheard of. Conditions and circumstances have changed. We may have succeeded in pushing up the expected life span of people over recent decades, but at what price? Yes, we have brought about many changes and most certainly many of them are improvements, but we have moved from our gentle and natural ways of healing towards the scientific and chemical ways, which are so much more harsh and drastic, and the side-effects are often too high a price to pay.

The message I wish to convey can be found in the simple Maori saying, with which I intend to close this book; it is a message for young and old alike:

*Mou te thi ete,*
*te tai po.*

*For you the morning tide,*
*For me the evening tide.*